Medical Anecdotes and

T0229434

Myocardial Medley

Edited by Ian R. Gray

from contributions submitted by members of
the General Practitioner Writers Association

Radcliffe Medical Press · Oxford

©1990 Radcliffe Medical Press Ltd
15 Kings Meadow, Ferry Hinksey Road, Oxford OX2 0DP

British Library Cataloguing in Publication Data
Gray, Ian
Myocardial medley. (Medical anecdotes and humour)
1. Jokes in English, 1945–Special subjects: medicine–
Anthologies
I. Title II. Series
828'.91402'080356

ISBN 1 870905 36 9

Any reference to products in this book does not imply endorsement by the editor or authors. Any reference to named, living individuals is purely coincidental.

Photoset by Enset, Midsomer Norton, Avon
Printed and bound by Billings, Worcester

Contents

Preface   vii

Acknowledgements   ix

1 Introduction

The Heart of the Matter   1
PETER BURKE, *Southampton*

What is Typically British?   2
CHRISTOPHER J. BARRATT, *Northwich*

Jack Sprat   3
MARIE CAMPKIN, *London*

Little Miss Muffage   4
MARIE CAMPKIN, *London*

2 Tools of the Trade

The Heart and Circulation: a Glossary   5
STEPHEN HEAD, *Newark*

A Scope for all Reasons   18
JOHN TAYLOR, *Lichfield*

In Praise of the Two-second Stethoscope   22
JOHN WOODWARD, *Sidcup*

Now you Hear it, Now you Don't   24
B.T. MARSH, *Chalfont St Peter*

CVS Made Easy   25
LAURENCE KNOTT, *East Barnet*

Initial Impressions   27
DAVID HASLAM, *Huntingdon*

Me and My ECG Machine   28
RONALD MULROY, *Wakefield*

3 Cardiac Arrest

Arrested Development   36
  KEITH HOPCROFT, *Basildon*

Perks of the Job   44
  P.J. SOUTH, *Frittenden*

Mary, Mary   52
  MARIE CAMPKIN, *London*

Humpty Dumpty   52
  MARIE CAMPKIN, *London*

4 Recollections

An Education of Hearts   53
  ANN WHITEHEAD, *London*

Houseman Hearts, or Tickers to Remember   66
  JOHN MACLEOD, *Isle of North Uist*

The Marsh Quality of Life Profile   72
  B.T. MARSH, *Chalfont St Peter*

Cardiac *faux pas*   76
  ROBIN HULL, *Birmingham*

Sing a Song   78
  MARIE CAMPKIN, *London*

5 Medical History

Directly from his Inmost Heart   79
  E. MEINHARDT, *Oxford*

6 Short Stories from General Practice

The Enchantment of George:
a Ghost Story from General Practice   88
  JOHN WOODWARD, *Sidcup*

Prentice Finch   98
  JOHN WOODWARD, *Sidcup*

Mary Ella and the Slipper: a Modern Fairy Tale   107
  JILL THISTLETHWAITE, *Luddendon*

Hypertension 111
JAMES HENRY PITT-PAYNE, *Beckenham*

Hearts 117
SAUL MILLER, *Cardiff*

The Private Clinic 119
MARIE CAMPKIN, *London*

Little Boy Blue 119
MARIE CAMPKIN, *London*

Georgy Porgy 120
MARIE CAMPKIN, *London*

Index 121

Preface

The medical profession has always produced a number of authors in addition to those whose writing was confined to medical subjects. For many of these their writing has nothing to do with their medical training or professional experience, although the special relationship between doctor and patient in times of illness and distress may have enriched their understanding of people and their behaviour. The manuscripts from which this anthology is selected were submitted by family doctors in a competition for humorous writing, and they all have something to do with the heart. Since all the contributions are written by doctors and are connected, however loosely, with their practice, many are based, sometimes closely, on personal experiences. This may explain why the writings, although always interesting and often quite fascinating, are not for the most part humorous; there is comedy but little comicality. With heart disease patient and doctor are both coming to terms with something that may be life-threatening. After a professional career devoted to cardiology, I cannot remember many situations which, even in retrospect, were entertaining to any of those concerned.

This collection therefore has a different flavour to its predecessor *Alimentary, My Dear Doctor*. It is a little more serious, and the pieces selected are often longer; more essays and short stories and fewer anecdotes. The quality of the writing is as high. The emphasis on comedy rather than tragedy excludes the bitter and the unpleasant; characters are more often agreeable than otherwise; and strangely, for the writings of doctors, there is hardly a mention of money or of politics!

I am sure that readers will gain as much enjoyment from sharing the thoughts and experiences of these doctor/writers as I have.

IAN R. GRAY
Warwick

Acknowledgements

R adcliffe Medical Press would like to thank the members of the General Practitioner Writers Association for contributing so enthusiastically to the competition on which this book is based.

The cartoons were drawn by Bernard Cookson whose work appears regularly in both the medical and national press.

1
Introduction

The Heart of the Matter

This is a topic close to my heart. From ancient times the heart has been placed on the ladder of nobility between the stomach and the brain. It is the organ of love, loyalty and passion. With an Anglo-Saxon nose for the prosaic, it was Harvey who reduced it to the humble status of a pump. Yet even the English, much less the hearty Latins, find it hard not to see it as much more. It remains at the core of our being – it is the true self to which everything else is a mere trifle in more metaphors than any other part of the body.

In imagery the composition and place of the heart is almost infinitely variable. Hearts can be of gold, of stone, of glass, of a lion, or even – in football parlance – of Midlothian. The heart can be in the mouth, in the hand, in the boots, on one's sleeve, in the right place, left in San Francisco, buried at Wounded Knee, or even just in it. Where the anatomists are really left standing is in finding esoterica such as the strings, cockles, portals and bottom of the heart.

At heart is where the old and young and where politicians tell us, in their quest for our hearts and minds, that they have our best interests. It is in our heart of hearts that we doubt them, particularly when they put their hand on their heart and recite by heart their heartening rhetoric.

The condemned man eats a hearty meal, and yet heartily is the way we like to laugh. Tabloid press stories range from heartrending to heartwarming; we can be in good heart or heartsick and our patients – using the newest buzz-word – can give us heartsink. Thanks range from heartfelt to half-hearted.

Heartsearching is a time-honoured activity. When a man looks into his heart what can he find? Heartache, heartburn, a heavy, lonely or noble heart, or, for that matter, no heart at all.

The heart is not always well treated in language. As well as being broken, it can be eaten out, pierced with an arrow, crossed, made to miss a beat or stand still, or put crossways.

The litany could go on and on forever, but really – I haven't got the heart.

PETER BURKE
Southampton

What is Typically British?

What about deckchairs on Skegness beach? Or queueing for fish and chips? Where else would you see the odd spectacle of Pantomine, where men dress as women and women pretend to be men, while sensible adults from the audience shout 'He's behind you', and other silly phrases. We all recognise that particular lunacy which sets we British apart from other nations, don't we (Oh no, we don't)?

But what of our people, aren't they unique too? Where else can you observe a creature like our British Fat Slob? Due to extensive Euro-cloning this individual is fast becoming extinct. His appearance has never concerned him. Short hair, style unchanged for years. Favourite clothes: at home, vest and braces; when out, cardigan; at the seaside, perhaps knotted handkerchief and rolled-up trousers. For six nights a week he can be found, with his friends, in the saloon bar in the local pub. He drinks mild ale and smokes Park Drive or Woodbine cigarettes. The conversation always concerns football managers, union affairs, the quality of the ale or 'the wife's' family. Favourite expressions are 'I'll just have a swift half', or 'I could murder a pint'.

On Saturday night he takes 'the wife' to the sing-song at the same pub. He is a chauvinist, but he is not aware of it: it just comes naturally.

The house is *her* territory. He would never interfere by offering to perform certain tasks, such as cooking or washing up, or even more definitely dusting, ironing or hoovering. He has never given even a moment's thought to his way of life . . . but all this is changing.

Health clubs, jogging, low cholesterol diets, don't do this, eat more of that; where is it all leading? 'The wife' is starting to nag about his weight. She isn't cooking chips any longer; no eggs and bacon for breakfast, no butter, no cream cakes. He was always that size; why, his father was heavy boned and his brother has a large frame. He doesn't need exercise, he walks to the pub every night, doesn't he?

But the pub has been revamped, the saloon is now a wine bar/bistro. You can't get mild or Park Drive any more; grown men drink cissy lager or fizzy water.

Rather like the dinosaur gradually lurching his last in the swamps, the British Fat Slob is dying out. His natural habitat is shrinking. Where is he safe? Even at the doctor's surgery he can't hide. Why, 'the doctor's' is supposed to be a refuge: the affable family friend, perhaps a little grumpy, but always there with a cough bottle. He didn't want his blood pressure checked or his cholesterol done. What difference does it make that his father died of a heart attack; that was years ago?

The world must be going mad. He knew that when they told him to alter his lifestyle. It isn't a style, an act, something to swop and change – it is him, not his way of life. Isn't it?

CHRISTOPHER J. BARRATT
Northwich

Jack Sprat

Jack Sprat would eat no fat,
His wife would eat no lean,
He's still alive at eighty-five,
She died at seventeen

MARIE CAMPKIN
London

Little Miss Muffage

Little Miss Muffage,
Needing more roughage,
Gave up her curds and whey,
With F-Plan she's trimmer
And fitter and slimmer
And spiders retreat in dismay

MARIE CAMPKIN
London

2
Tools of the Trade

R eaders unfamiliar with the heart and heart disease may find some of the later contributions easier to understand after studying the glossary of terms and the description of the aids to diagnosis set out in this section.

The Heart and Circulation: a Glossary

A-type personality

Ask most people the cause of heart attacks and they will reply 'stress'. In fact, there is little scientific evidence for this. However, tense, impatient people who are always getting worked up because things are behind schedule do seem to be at greater risk than gentle, relaxed souls.

Considering how tense, impatient people tend to make life hell for others besides themselves, maybe they deserve it. Apart from the stress they are likely to have an unhealthy lifestyle, grabbing cigarettes and junk food amid their horrid, high-pressure lives.

Angina

Angina is a fancy word for pain, and angina pectoris are two fancy words for pain felt in the chest. Doctors use these terms for pain arising from the heart despite (a) most chest pain having other causes and (b) pain from the heart often being felt in other places like the arms, neck and belly.

The pain is caused when the heart muscle tissue is short of oxygen and says 'ouch'. The most common cause is atheroma (*see* next page). Though sometimes serious, some people lead a long and happy life despite the occasional twinge.

Anticoagulants

These are drugs that 'thin the blood', that is, make it less likely to clot. Certain types of heart patient take these, especially where there is a risk of blood clots forming in the heart itself (and you do not need a medical degree to realise that this is a bad thing).

Patients on these drugs must be careful what they drink and need regular blood checks which help to remind them how ill they are and how much care they need to take of themselves. Not surprisingly, they often do very well.

Arrhythmia

The word rhythm prefixed by the Greek 'a' meaning absent (cf., amoral: having no morals). Doctors therefore use this word to describe people who do have a heart rhythm, albeit irregular. Doctors call people who do not have a heart rhythm dead people (*see* cardiac arrest).

Arteries

These are the vessels which carry the blood away from the heart. The blood travels in pulses in time with the heartbeat, and this pulse can be felt. Doctors take the pulse to check its strength and rhythm. They also take the pulse as a gesture of kindness and comfort to patients. If a doctor feels that some examination of the patient is expected, but cannot think of anything much to do, a quick check of the pulse always reassures.

Atheroma

This is the build-up of fatty tissue, furring up the blood vessels. When it occurs in the heart it causes angina and heart attacks. This is the most common cause of death in most Western countries. The fat starts to be laid down in teenage years; cigarette smoking and an unhealthy lifestyle make it worse. Health education is mainly aimed at preventing atheroma.

Atrium (plural atria)

The two upper chambers of the heart are called the left atrium and the right atrium. On a chest X-ray the films are always displayed so that the left atrium is on the right (as you look at it) and the right on the left. This is one of the little tricks doctors use to maintain their professional mystique from so-called intelligent laymen.

The atria receive the blood returning to the heart through the veins. The blood sits around there until it gets pushed through into the ventricles to be pumped off again. The atria are not very exciting bits and often in transplant operations they do not bother to replace them because they are so boring.

B-type personalities

These are the sort of people who seem less likely to get heart trouble. They never seem to be under pressure, ignore deadlines and do not get worked-up or excited.

They might express fulsome gratitude for this great good fortune – only they can not be bothered.

Cardiac arrest

This is when the heart stops beating. If the cause is in the heart it can sometimes be put right provided it is done quickly. Otherwise it means the same as being dead. If you are planning a cardiac arrest, choose a place where skilled help is at hand, usually in or near a major hospital. Other good places are swimming pools (where the attendants are trained in resuscitation) and golf courses (which are often teeming with doctors).

Treatment of cardiac arrest is simple. Someone batters the patient around the chest while someone else performs mouth-to-mouth breathing. When the patient arrives at a defibrillator (or vice versa) this is used to make the heart beat again. If that does not work various drugs are tried, plus further electric shocks from the defibrillator.

Busy junior doctors man the cardiac arrest teams and spend many hours running round hospitals to people who have arrested in order to save the patient's life and their own: they have so little time off, this is the only healthy exercise they get.

Cardiac neurosis

Nervous preoccupation with the heart leading to disability despite normal examination findings (and maybe a pretty ropey history too). This is far less fashionable than it used to be, maybe because people who complain enough are likely to end up having various nasty tests done (such as tubes shoved through their blood vessels into the heart) while they are still awake.

People with nervous trouble are advised to front-up and deal with the real problem. People who wish to feign illness will do well to stick to back pain and dizzy turns.

Cardiac sphincter

This is the valve between the bottom of the gullet (the tube from the throat through which various things are swallowed) and the stomach. It is meant to allow food and drink to pass downward but prevent stomach acid and other stomach contents passing upwards. When the whole thing goes crazy and allows massive backflow of stomach contents vomiting occurs.

The adjective 'cardiac' means of course 'pertaining to the heart'; nevertheless, the cardiac sphincter has about as much to do with the heart as the left big toe – it just happens to be closer.

Cardiologists

These are physicians who specialise in heart disease. They have specialised in internal medicine, which means that they do lots of tests and then prescribe pills (cf., surgeons).

There are not many cardiologists in Britain and they tend to stick together in a few regional centres. Most people with heart disease who see a specialist see a local physician who is not quite that specialised. Considering that a lot of people with suspected heart trouble turn out instead to have diseases of the stomach, spine, muscles, etc., this is quite a good idea, really.

Cardio-thoracic surgeons

The hell and glory boys of heart disease, these are the people who chop out leaky valves and blocked coronary arteries and replace them with new ones. They tend to work closely with cardiologists and usually only operate if a cardiologist asks them.

Obviously, if things are not that bad, major and potentially hazardous surgery will not be necessary. On the other hand, if people are very ill they are unlikely to survive a major operation anyway. It follows that only a carefully selected group of patients are given operations: people whose hearts are bad, but not *that* bad.

Circulation

The blood circulates around the blood vessels and heart. It travels in a particular direction: from the right ventricle it passes to the lungs to pick up oxygen; then it passes through the left atrium into the left ventricle from where it is pumped round the body to return to the right ventricle via the right atrium. It took early doctors centuries to work this out: though it seems quite obvious now.

Claudication

This is a pain felt in the legs when walking due to atheroma blocking the arteries. It is like angina of the legs. For a non-smoker it is a rarity. Most patients get better by stopping smoking and practising walking. Some need surgery to unblock the vessels.

The word is derived from the Emperor Claudius, who was considered to be a 'pain'.

Coronary arteries

These are the blood vessels which supply blood to the heart muscle itself. They branch off from the main artery, the aorta, just outside the heart and wander back down and round the heart muscle. They were called coronary arteries because the early anatomy people thought they looked like a crown. The reaction of most medical students when dissecting a heart is that they look nothing like a crown and that hallucinogenic drugs have probably been around universities longer than most people assume.

Coronary by-pass graft

This is the deceptively simple operation where nasty old blocked vessels are replaced by new ones, often by taking veins from the leg. An alternative is to leave the old ones in but scrape all the nasty furr off their insides. Like most surgery this sounds easier than it is. It is worth remembering this use of leg veins for life-saving operations, especially if a varicose veins operation is contemplated. Once they have been stripped the chance of a good vein graft to save your life can be ruined.

On operating lists the operation is often acronymised to CABAGE: a useful reminder to the anaesthetist that the patient's brain needs to be carefully protected during the operation.

Coronary care units

These are very high-tech wards where people with heart attacks are sometimes nursed. You can always tell how ill you are by seeing if you have more wires and tubes attached to your body than the patient in the next bed. Also the various bits of gadgetry tend to click every time your heart beats, which means that you are not at risk of dying without noticing.

The benefits of these units are not as clear cut as might be thought. Some patients do very well staying at home after their heart attack: they certainly have more peace and quiet. Being surrounded by other people with the same trouble as you has major shortcomings: especially when (as is sadly often the case) they keep dying.

Coronary thrombosis

This is what so-called intelligent laymen, show-offs and snobs call a heart attack. Most doctors call a heart attack a myocardial infarction. A few charming and wonderful doctors call it a heart attack.

Never say 'coronary thrombosis' – it is silly, pretentious and not even current medical usage.

Dextrocardia

This is a rare condition where the heart and the bits attached to it are the wrong way round, like a mirror image. As a result the heartbeat is felt best on the right of the chest; there are lots more subtle differences any competent fourth-year medical student will spot – if they know what they are looking for.

Dextrocardia is no threat to health, it all works just the same. However, if these people ever go to hospital for whatever reason they will be mobbed by students and junior doctors who have never seen a case. Stoical sorts, who can put up with that sort of thing, often turn up at medical school to be used as subjects for students to practise on in their exams. This teaches the students a very important lesson – to be nice to people. The dextrocardiac patient can tell the student what the findings should be and will do so (ensuring the student passes) if the student seems a decent sort. Moral – there is more to good doctoring than sound theoretical knowledge.

The mischievous dextrocardiac can have endless fun at life insurance medicals and the like.

Diet and heart disease

Certain foods seem to make heart disease more likely. Sugars disturb healthy metabolism, increasing the risk of diabetes, which in turn increases the risk of heart trouble. Fats, dairy food and animal protein (which always has a high fat content) increase the deposit of fat in the arteries which causes heart attacks. Starchy foods are fattening, and obesity is bad for the heart. Salt and alcohol increase the blood pressure and raise the cholesterol level.

Heart disease is rare among fruit bats with anorexia nervosa.

Drugs and the heart

Several different types of drug are used to treat heart disease, and there are hundreds of drugs altogether. Below is a brief review of the more common groups. Each drug has a generic name plus one or more trade names, which are different. All this makes it very difficult for ordinary people to figure just what they are taking and why. If you want to take this seriously, ask your doctor what type of drugs you are on. You might be told.

(a) Beta-blockers. These drugs relax the heart, slow the heart rate, lower the blood pressure and sometimes steady the heart rhythm. They can make you a bit tired but it has been proved that they improve the performance of cello players. Their generic names usually end in -olol (goodness knows why). If you are on beta-blockers you would be well advised to take up the cello: it will take your mind off your heart trouble, and you can do it sitting down which should not strain things too much.

(b) Nitrates. These drugs are used to ease the pain of angina. They are thought to do this by relaxing the blood vessels. They sometimes lower the blood pressure, but are not really meant to. Some are tablets to be sucked or chewed, some swallowed, some sprayed in the mouth and some stuck on the skin as a patch. The most widely used nitrate is glyceryl trinitrate, which is none other than the explosive TNT. However, for treating heart disease it is only used in low doses, and never with a fuse.

(c) Calcium blockers. These lower the blood pressure, relieve angina and help steady the heart rhythm. Their names tend to end in -pine.

(d) Diuretics. These increase the loss of fluid from the body which helps heart failure. They also tend to lower the blood pressure. In the good old days the same effect was achieved by blood-letting. It might be fashionable to knock the drug industry but this must be a step in the right direction.

ECG (or electrocardiogram)

This is a machine that provides an electrical tracing of the heart. Patients are often reassured when they have one, and it is normal. This is wrong because people can have angina or even a heart attack despite a perfectly normal ECG. Before these expensive machines, doctors checked the heart by listening to it with a stethoscope. ECGs became fashionable at about the time medical students and young doctors took to going to discos and playing loud music – they are now too deaf to rely on their own ears for diagnosis.

The heart

The heart is about the size of the clenched fist. It sits in the chest just behind the breast bone and a little lopsided to the left. On either side of it there is a lung. Below it is the diaphragm; above it all the plumbing bits like the big arteries and veins. Behind the heart is the gullet, some more blood vessels and the spine.

Your heart should beat about 3500 million times during your lifetime.

Heartburn

As the name would suggest, heartburn has absolutely nothing to do with the heart.

It is a feeling of burning discomfort felt around where the heart happens to be. In fact the pain arises from the gullet. Heartburn occurs when stomach acid (which is a wonderful thing in the right place) leaks backwards up into the gullet (the wrong place). Here it burns the lining causing the symptom (*see* cardiac sphincter).

Heart failure

This term is used to mean many different things, the common feature being that the heart is not pumping as well as it should. Treating heart failure is much easier and more effective than it used to be. The most effective drugs are diuretics which make the patient pass more water. Inducing medical students to try to explain how running to the loo can take the strain off the failing heart is a source of endless amusement during oral examinations.

Heart valves

There are four valves in the heart, and they are like valves anywhere else: their job is to ensure that the blood flows in one direction only. Valves can leak, which means that the blood can flow backwards, or be too tight, which means that it cannot flow forwards as easily as it should.

Trouble with valves can cause murmurs. Badly affected valves can be surgically replaced with new ones, although these often make more noise than the old ones. Patients have been known to complain that their new valve was so noisy it disturbed their sleep.

Hypertension

This is high blood pressure. A common condition, most cases have no known cause. Being fat and drinking a lot of alcohol make it worse. Untreated it causes strokes, heart and kidney problems. Usually, sensible living and one or two tablets a day control the condition.

Doctors call high blood pressure hypertension and low blood pressure hypotension; they often defend their jargon by saying it makes what they say less confusing: perhaps this one needs some further thought.

Hypotension

This is low blood pressure. Apart from a few very rare diseases it is a problem in older people whose blood pressure falls when they stand up. This happens because the lining of the blood vessels becomes stiff and lagged up with age and so cannot respond quickly to the changing effects of gravity when they move from lying to standing. This is not the origin of the term 'old lag', although perhaps it should have been.

Murmurs

Most people have two heart sounds. Some have more and these extra sounds are called murmurs. Most are quite harmless and innocent: with all that blood rushing around the odd bit of noise is hardly surprising.

Sometimes a murmur is caused by a hole in the heart or trouble with the heart valves: this might be serious.

If you, or someone you love, is found to have a murmur at a routine medical examination or accidentally when the doctor was doing something else, it is more than likely to be nothing to worry about. Serious murmurs mean serious heart disease and if the person's health is generally alright nothing is likely to be amiss.

The biggest problem with having a murmur is that medical students and young doctors are quite likely to want to listen to it. Queues of eager white-coated persons gather at the foot of your hospital bed (never mind that you are only there to have your piles seen to). If you have a murmur, do not like hordes of strange people, and need to go into hospital – go private.

Myocardial infarction

This is what doctors call a heart attack. There is a blockage of blood flow in the coronary vessels so that part of the heart muscle dies. People having heart attacks get severe pain somewhere round the chest, and turn clammy. Urgent medical care is essential.

Do not have your attack sitting at home: you will wait a while to see if it eases and try a dose of indigestion medicine or something else. Have your heart attack in a supermarket or on a busy street. Someone will realise what is happening even if you do not and help will soon be at hand.

Sometimes people with heart attacks have no symptoms, or very different symptoms (like giddiness or feeling faint). There is often nothing out of the ordinary to be found on examining a patient with a heart attack. Nevertheless, many of these patients are diagnosed, which just goes to show why training a doctor takes so long but why it is probably worth it.

Treatment of myocardial infarction involves relieving the pain, maybe trying to dissolve the blockage with drugs, and watching for complications such as heart failure or disorders of heart rhythm.

Pacemakers

Sometimes the heart beats too slowly and an artificial pacemaker can be fitted to keep the heart rate correct; these machines are now far more reliable than in the past. Some are powered by a small nuclear reactor and they must be removed before people are cremated: otherwise they can explode leaving nuclear contamination around the Chapel of Rest.

Palpitations

Technically, and in common language, an awareness of the heartbeat. Most people most of the time are unaware of their heartbeat. Most people some of the time are (after vigorous exercise for example), but would never dream of giving it a second thought, let alone seeing a doctor.

People who see a doctor with palpitations are therefore fascinating, but their hearts are probably boringly normal.

Sphygmomanometer

This is the machine doctors use to measure blood pressure. If you ever have cause to suspect that your doctor has been drinking on duty (sadly not an unknown situation), get him to check your blood pressure then ask him what the thing he is using is called.

Stethoscope

The doctor's badge; patients often wonder what the doctor listening to their heart hears. Not much: two heart sounds, rarely a murmur, and that is about all. If the heart sounds are not there you are dead. All the common heart trouble seen by family doctors does not change the way the heart sounds at all.

Then why listen? First, to impress on the patient that the job has been properly done. Secondly, to impress colleagues by mentioning anything unusual if referring the patient. Thirdly, for the reason people climb mountains: so long as Mount Everest is in the Himalayas mountaineers will climb it; and so long as doctors walk round with stethoscopes dangling from their necks patients will have their hearts listened to.

Strokes

Strokes are to the brain what heart attacks are to the the heart. A blood vessel becomes blocked, damaged or bleeds leaving part of the brain tissue to die due to lack of oxygen. Medical students and ambulance men sometimes call strokes CVAs (cerebro-vascular accidents). This is a bit pretentious: *see* coronary thrombosis. No one calls strokes apoplexy any more, which seems a pity – a nice old-fashioned term.

Syncope

Pronounced 'sin copy'. Means a faint. People faint when there is not enough blood reaching the brain to keep them conscious. Standing for long periods, being tired or hungry or upset make it more likely, as do things like a touch of 'flu. The blood pressure falls when people faint and fainting is more common in people with low blood pressure anyway. Since this same low blood pressure will make them less likely to acquire heart trouble or strokes, they should maybe be more congratulated than diagnosed.

The treatment of syncope is to lie the patient horizontally so that the blood can flow straight instead of uphill from the heart to the brain. Syncope is dangerous when this cannot happen, such as in a telephone box or very cramped toilet: people who tend to faint would do well to eat a hearty meal before using either.

Veins

Veins tend to be the forgotten part of the circulation. Hearts are glamorous, arteries are exciting, veins are veins. This is a pity: they are a vital and complex part of the body. A clot forming in a vein is a serious emergency (it can move to the lung and cause death). Varicose veins are unsightly, occasionally dangerous and operations for them are intricate and challenging; but if you want to be famous best stick to heart transplants.

Ventricles

These are the other two chambers of the heart (see atrium). The right ventricle is so-called because it is in front of the left ventricle. The left ventricle is the largest and most powerful of the heart's chambers, as it has to provide the contraction to send the blood right round the body.

STEPHEN HEAD
Newark

A Scope for all Reasons

Have you ever asked yourself why doctors carry stethoscopes? Well, probably not, since the answer seems so obvious. To listen to the heart of course, or occasionally, if it is one of those funny champagne-glass-shaped-ones, the pulsating womb. But why such a simple device in this technological age, since nowadays they have all the advances modern science can provide to enhance their diagnostic skills?

They are able to examine almost every nook and cranny of the human frame without getting the hands dirty at all. Notwithstanding the claims of some 'alternative' physicians who can tell all, they say, from a study of the soles of the feet, the modern doctor can, if he wants to, traverse the bowels from end to end, hardly touching the sides, and can see into lungs, look at livers, observe ovaries and the goings-on inside them and much, much more, with their patient's hair hardly turning at all. Indeed, during many such diagnostic occasions, the observations may actually be shared with the operatee by means of dual eyepieces or TV monitors.

'Scoping' is not confined to the visual spectrum either, since we can now make observations (which is what the word means) by using many other modalities as well. There are devices to pick up sound waves of one frequency or another being bounced off things that should or should not be there. Machines are available to pick up electrical charges that are passing through heart muscle or brain cells.

Despite all this fancy equipment, however, the instrument that is still most commonly used and carried around by doctors is the good old stethoscope. The truth is, of course, that the 'scope, or 'tubes', may be carried for a variety of different reasons, some of which are certainly not clinical ones, and some of which may also depend upon the doctor's seniority and speciality, or his/her motives, ulterior or otherwise.

The day the young medical student passed the second MB examination, after two years of anatomy and other subjects, should have been one to be remembered. Well, it should have been, but it rarely was, because it usually took a few days to get the brain cells focusing again after the celebration. When recovery had occurred though it was apparent to most that they had now been translated into another world populated by live people, rather than dissecting-room remains. One way of marking this passage was to buy a stethoscope. The instrument became a badge, a talisman even, the carrying of which announced to one and all that they were proper doctors, and now worthy of more respect than hitherto afforded, particularly by the likes of student nurses. (Senior nurses or ward sisters were not that easily fooled but then we were not trying to impress them.)

Fortunately, the aforesaid student nurses did not usually know the real definition of the new 'badge': stethoscope means after all, when literally translated, 'to observe the breast'. Mind you, if male, and by carrying one this latter goal was also achieved, who was to complain? It was a commonly known fact in those heady days that one's desirability as a potential mate increased in proportion to the nearness of qualification, and possession of a stethoscope was one step in the right direction. Initially, we usually had the thing dangling around our necks at all times, apart from when in the pub or playing rugby. Where this display was deemed to be rather vulgar, such as on trains or buses, we made sure that the earpieces protruded from the pocket and were plain for all to see. We assumed that most people would not know that we, as yet, could not tell a heart sound from a bowel sound, since we were now addressed as 'that young doctor'.

So there we are, to start with; two good reasons for having a stethoscope that had nothing to do with its proper use; that is, to impress student nurses and to win more respect from the public, which included 'our' patients.

There then followed a rather painful period, which in my day was called an 'introductory course to clinical medicine'. Apart from having to learn to take a patient history of such detail that carrying it about afterwards would induce a rupture, we were instructed in the art of the physical examination. The scenes depicted in the film *Doctor in the House* (J. Arthur Rank, made during the 1950s), where discomfiture was visited upon luckless students by the morning-coated consultant, were as nothing in comparison to the actual events. 'Is that a stethoscope I see, Mr Smith? Well, come and show us all how you use it to make a diagnosis'. For a while we tried to pretend that we did not own one, and deliberately left them behind. During one such encounter one of my friends, in a fit of panic, was somehow persuaded to come forward and place his instrument upon the thigh of a young man, which was bulging with a swelling. He had not been able to recognise the mass, which turned out to be a lipoma (a simple fatty swelling), and in desperation said that he would like to listen to it with his stethoscope first, before proffering a diagnosis. After a prolonged silence, associated with much smirking from the rest of us and a rather unpleasant leer from the consultant, the truth was revealed. On every occasion thereafter my friend was offered an opportunity to 'auscultate', whether the object was an ingrowing toe-nail, a hernia or a varicose vein. After qualification I am sure that the first thing he did was to throw his 'scope away, because in due course he became a world renowned immunologist and did not have to use one. By then, of course, he did not have to impress student nurses, either.

Flaunting a stethoscope then, may not always be advantageous, but there are occasions when having one about might be helpful. For instance, if left casually draped across the front seat of the car, one might be able to unduly influence police officers. Once, during a time when I was demonstrating anatomy, and far away from clinical work, I had the misfortune to run into the back of another car at a road junction. No real damage was done, but the impact brought busy rush hour traffic to a standstill and, of course, with this arrived a curious policeman. He leaned into the car, about to be sarcastic, when he saw my 'scope. There was a pause, and then . . .' well, Sir, shall we just say that your brakes were not as good as his'. End of conversation. The owner of the assaulted car was not quite so polite, but at any event the Law was no longer interested. There are disadvantages to this wanton display, of course. Villains are very observant and on the basis of stethoscope means doctor, *ergo* possibility of drugs on board, doctors' cars are much more vulnerable to theft. What is more, not all policemen are so naïve as to believe that a doctor is on an errand of mercy when travelling with stethoscope exposed: I was once followed right into the hospital's operating suite by one such cynic, who doubted the veracity of my stated need to go through a traffic light at red; I was only saved by the red line on the theatre floor, over which he was not pemitted to pass.

A forensic pathologist of my acquaintance, who to my certain knowledge had not seen a live patient since his medical student days, could always get away with his affirmative answer when challenged for some driving misdemeanour. 'Are you saying, Sir, that you are on a life or death matter?' The stethoscope again.

It is obvious that the carrying of the 'scope still imparts some sense of superiority, since nowadays not only doctors do this but many nurses, as well. Modern fashion dictates that they should be casually draped across the shoulders. This is fair enough when nurses are doing some of the doctoring, as in midwifery or in Intensive Therapy units, but in North America all nurses have taken up the habit.

Which takes me to my last point. There is one group of the medical profession who not only do not want to pretend to be doctors, but who would positively resent being mistaken for ordinary doctors in any circumstance: I refer, of course, to surgeons.

There are many reasons for this, the most important being that most surgeons know nothing about vulgar things like heart sounds in the first place, and much embarrassment may thereby be avoided. In any event, where can a surgeon carry one, without spoiling the cut of the three-piece pinstripe?

There may be many reasons why the doctor hangs on to his stethoscope, but it may have absolutely nothing to do with the wellbeing, or otherwise, of your heart.

JOHN TAYLOR

Lichfield

In Praise of the Two-second Stethoscope

Times have changed. Days were when the frightened patient with chest pain could be dismissed with two seconds of pressure from the stethoscope over the praecordium 'Thank you, doctor', he would stammer, his eyes brimming with tears of gratitude and out he would go into his own world with no more cares on his shoulders.

The first gust of the wind of change blew in the cardiograph. 'Are you quite sure my heart's all right, doctor? Shouldn't I have an ECG?' So, ever-mindful of his patients' needs, the family doctor splashed out a thousand or more totally irretrievable pounds and began to run off a succession of useless tracings for which he received the approbation of the incumbent of the Elephant and Castle but not a penny in reimbursement. Of course, the patient was not initially aware of the fact that a resting ECG does not exclude coronary heart disease, so for a while his doctor could use the machine much as he had previously used his stethoscope, but with inestimably greater panache. Alas, it could not last.

Someone on a television 'soap' filtered in the knowledge that ECGs in the doctor's surgery are nearly as much a waste of time as listening to the heart; so the expensive electronic hardware is now probably redundant in primary care. Nevertheless, there is no doubt that every good practice will continue to equip itself with the latest cardiograph machine as it does with computers or emergency resuscitation trolleys, because that is what every good practice does, isn't it?

'What I really want, doctor, is a treadmill test'.

'Of course, Mr Smith. There is a nine-month waiting list on the NHS, but doubtless your firm will pay for a private appointment tomorrow'. And off the patient goes for the first fifteen minutes of exercise he has had in the last ten years.

Then there was a *British Medical Journal* leader which suggested that treadmill tests produced unreliable results. It has reached the ears of Monsieur Hominrue and his reactions have been entirely predictable. He will waste no further time in the foothills. He demands to be placed at once on the summit of the mountain of health care. 'This pain in my chest, doctor – send me to a top Harley Street specialist. I'm sure I need an angiogram'.

He presents two fallacies. First, a top Harley Street specialist is simply a doctor who lives at the upper end of the thoroughfare. Harley Street is an address, not a qualification. Secondly, he does not require an angiogram.

Modern cardiac technology has produced its own human wreckage, and Britain cannot afford the bill. It is time to bring back the two-second stethoscope.

JOHN WOODWARD

Sidcup

Now you Hear it, Now you Don't

Did you know that the twenty-fourth edition of *Dorland's Illustrated Medical Dictionary, 1967* lists 75 different heart murmurs? No? Well, nor did I. I'll bet that you also did not know that there are 71 in the twenty-seventh edition of 1988. The trouble is, many of them have changed, and for the worse if you aks me; not only that, the definition of murmur has altered from the pleasant evocative 'gentle blowing ausculatory sound' reminding one of a sun-kissed walk on the Downs to 'an ausculatory sound, benign or pathologic, particularly a periodic sound of short duration of cardiac or vascular origin' more redolent of an expensive and disagreeable appointment in Harley Street.

Never again will we hear Bright's murmur, so beautifully described as a *bruit de cuir neuf*, whatever that is. No Eustace Smith's murmur, or Fisher's murmer, or Fraentzel's murmur. Gone too is the lapping murmur, Makin's murmur and the metallic murmur. Oh pray for the return of the nun's murmur, also called, and don't ask me why, *bruit de diable* and Parrot's murmur – of whom it could be said he must be as sick as a . . . At least the reduplication murmur has been rumbled, as has the spontaneous murmur, but feel sad for the loss of the *bruit de moulin*: the water-wheel murmur.

And what have we gained? Rubbish. The basal diastolic murmur, the holosystolic murmur and the pansystolic murmur – no character in these murmurs, all Filofaxes and briefcases. The continuous, incidental and innocent murmurs are nothing to write home about, either. The cooing murmur is a weak attempt to get back to the good old days but what about the diamond-shaped murmur? Who ever heard of a sound being diamond-shaped? The only new ones you can really roll around the tongue are Cruveilheir – Baumgarten's murmur – now, there is something worth listening for; Hamman's murmur – a crunching sound heard over the praecordium; and Carey Coombs murmur. Double-barrelled murmurs always sound much more important, don't you think?

However, there are still a few of the old gang about. Austin Flint's murmur is a posh one, in the same class as Graham

Steell's. Gibson and Still's murmurs are acceptable, but Duroziez's and Traube's murmurs sound a bit doubtful and Roger's murmur is definitely going too far, particularly as it might be involved with the poor nun's murmur. We can't get rid of the funnies such as the accidental murmur – I suppose that is the one we did not really hear, and the heart, cardiac and endocardial murmurs: tautology, if I ever heard it. The musical fraternity are still with us – the amphoric, bellows, crescendo, friction, humming-top, machinery, musical, organic (?), see-saw and to-and-fro murmurs provide us with the basis for a concerto by Gerard Hoffnung – but the hour-glass? Surely there must be some mistake?

I expect that in 20 years' time the list of murmurs will be even more anaemic (yes, that's still in) and uninteresting. Never mind, I'll be deaf by then and it won't matter. I never could decide whether a murmur was systolic or diastolic, and quite frankly I can't stand people who don't speak out properly, but twitter away like a sea-gull murmur. Pardon?

B.T. MARSH

Chalfont St Peter

CVS Made Easy

I have finally summoned up the courage to come out into the open and admit that I suffer from congenital blindness of the cardiovascular system. I am familiar with the ins and outs of the alimentary system, I am inspired by the respiratory system and I know the dorsum of the carpus like the back of my hand. The workings of that infernal pump and its series of graduated tubes, however, remains a mystery to me.

I am sure I cannot be the only one who, when reading articles about beta-receptors, smooth-muscled arterioles and sick sinuses might as well be perusing the Chinese telephone directory. Well, fear not, fellow sufferers, for help is at hand. In order to diagnose and treat disorders of the cardiovascular system, you do not actually have to understand it. Follow my simple method and you cannot go wrong.

First, feel the pulse at the patient's wrist. If it is there, you're onto a winner for a start. If it is regular, so much the better. If it is irregular, you must decide whether to differentiate between atrial flutter, ventricular extrasystoles and Wolff-Parkinson-White Syndrome, or whether you are simply going to call it irregular. Do the latter.

Auscultate the heart. There is no need to ask the patient to undress for this. I myself have become extremely adept at hearing a beating heart through a duffle coat, a Fair Isle jumper and several layers of thermal underwear. Do not worry about added fripperies such as split first and second sounds, heart murmurs and the like. If you do hear added sounds they are most likely to be the shuffling of feet in the waiting room.

Now, a couple of words about 4th and 5th Korotkoff sounds. Forget them. If you check the patient's blood pressure and can hear 1st, 2nd and 3rd Korotkoff sounds, quit while you are winning. If you cannot hear anything at all, go back to square one and check the patient's pulse. If you hear music, make sure you have picked up your stethoscope and not the headset of the patient's personal CD player.

At this point you will either suspect that something is up or that there is nothing wrong. If you find no abnormality on examination and the patient feels well, send them on their way. If you suspect that something is up and the patient feels ill, check whether they are taking tablets from their previous doctor. If they are, and you know the tablets, fiddle around with the dosage. If they are not, refer them to a physician.

That is about all there is to it, really. You will not win any prizes for contributions to the field of cardiovascular physiology, but you will get through Monday evening surgery with your dignity and sanity intact.

LAURENCE KNOTT
East Barnet

Initial Impressions

I have never understood what is wrong with words. They have been enough for most of the human race through the centuries; Shakespeare and Wordsworth found words to be sufficient for their purposes, and even the tabloid press includes a few words amongst the pictures. So why do hospital junior staff find them unnecessary?

You must have had letters like the one that arrived today concerning one of my patients. I had sent Mr Jackson into hospital with a suspected heart attack. He lived alone, had been hypertensive for some years, and not only did I have to ease his pain, order the ambulance, give him oxygen, hold his hand, utter reassuring words, inject atropine as he slipped into a dramatic bradycardia, sit him up and phone the hospital, but also find someone to care for his cat, turn off the cooker and lock up the house.

So how did he fare in hospital? The letter said it all.

'Dear Doctor', it started promisingly – but then those words were printed. '? MI, ECG NAD, BP OK, Rx ISQ, OPD 2/52'.

Sheer poetry. Where did this dreadful habit of abbreviating everything come from? Did the 'MI' refer to a myocardial infarction or mitral incompetence? Do women with an 'IUD' have an intra-uterine contraceptive device or an intra-uterine death? It does make something of a difference to your approach when you next see the patient. And what about those patients who are discharged from the super-specialist surgical units having had operations described as a '2-stage LCRFS'? How on earth does the average GP work out what an LCRFS might be, or even a humble one-stage version?

The rise of the dreadful 'query', as in '?MI' almost brings me out in a rash. I suppose it is just about bearable when written down, although I cannot understand why the question mark appears before the diagnosis. Does it sound too uncertain to put it afterwards? However, when the 'query' is used in speech it becomes plain absurd. To be phoned by a hospital doctor to be told that your patient has had a 'query heart attack' almost leaves him or her open to an official complaint to the English Usage Board (if there were one).

Oh, in case you are interested, Mr Jackson was OK after his '?MI' except that the hospital forgot to give him his TTOs for his BP and his CCF, along with the appointment for the OPD to see the SHO. His cat was fine.

DAVID HASLAM
Huntingdon

Me and My ECG Machine

To be perfectly honest, I do not understand machinery. I never have and I never will. Machines, especially the more intelligent ones, sense this in me and, throughout my life, have rejected me as I have rejected them.

It was not surprising then that I chose a career far removed from the mechanical sciences. Medicine was my choice, since it was concerned primarily with a warm biological mechanism that could, through natural, spontaneous appetites, maintain and reproduce itself. This same mechanism could tell you details of its own malfunction and – best of all – would often sort out its own problems, provided doctors allowed it. Unfortunately I entered Medical School at a time when medicine itself was beginning to suffer from a hypertrophy of machinery.

As soon as possible, I fled from the technical tyranny of hospital life to the vital pastures of general practice, but found I was unable to free myself entirely from the influence of the machine. I was, all too soon, aware of my naked vulnerability when practising medicine without technical support. Moreover, general practice was improving itself and the outward sign of this inward grace was the possession of an ECG machine. 'Own ECG' became an essential part of any advertisement of any vacancy in any practice worth its salt. It was obvious that no self-respecting GP could be without one – and I was, at least, self-respecting.

There were snags, of course, even if I could overcome my own fundamental unease in the face of machinery. For a start,

£200 was a lot of money to pay simply to resolve an occasional
clinical dilemma and to put a thin veneer of science on the mess
of everyday life. Then there was the difficulty with electricity.
My attitude to this magical substance owed more to James
Thurber than it did to science. I still have a gut feeling about
electricity being a fluid running through minute channels in
wires, leaking from empty plug sockets and dripping from
light fittings. An A-level in physics did nothing to convince me
otherwise. Curiously enough, I had no fears about interpret-
ing the actual tracings. After all, I had done my house jobs and
there were plenty of books.

I overcame the potential financial handicap by the simple
expedient of borrowing a redundant ECG machine from the
local cottage hospital. It was quite old and had a real leather
case, the faded lettering was in the Romanesque style and it
was heavy – probably about 30–40 lbs. At times the weight was
a disadvantage but, at least, it provided me with some much-
needed exercise. It was the plug that caused most trouble. The
hospital was built in the 15-amp era but many of the houses in
the practice had already converted to modern 13-amp plugs.
Many an hour I spent changing plugs at the bedside, for it was
some months before I was able to acquire a 13/15-amp adaptor.
My electrical kit accompanied me everywhere and was an essential part of my medical armamentarium. That is, providing
I could unzip the leather case. The zip had a mind of its own
but no fastener; – needed pliers for that. And somehow, there
was never enough jelly. It was always a mystery to me where
the jelly went. Fortunately, I came across a timely article by a
Bedfordshire physician in which he had scientifically explored
the efficacy of various household commodities as substitutes
for electrode jelly. Mayonnaise was undoubtedly the best so I
always carried some of my own, for one cannot always trust
patients in matters of taste. Being somewhat heavy laden as I
went about God's work, I found a broken handle on the case a
disadvantage, but I solved that problem easily enough with a
length of washing line, cunningly fashioned into a carrying
net.

Thus equipped, I set out to deliver the science of modern
medicine to the lucky people of Crigglethorpe. It was not long

before I had earned a reputation as a 'turn himself to anything' type of doctor, though remarkably few complimented me on my cardiology.

I soon discovered that there were more technical problems in using an ECG machine than I had imagined – and that after I had obtained access to the machine itself and the electricity. Most of these could be classified roughly under the heading of the 'AC Problem'. To tell the truth, I never did fathom the 'AC Problem', though, of course, I had my theories. The books were vague when describing the cause, but explicit in describing the effect – very rapid regular oscillations on the tracing. They were even more detailed when describing how to solve it. They reckoned it was all to do with electricity in the air and the earth's magnetism and similar scientific things. I followed their advice to the letter. First, I would turn the machine clockwise. If there was no response, I would then turn it anti-clockwise. This exercise proved a useful diversion to the patient with acute chest pain and distracted him from contemplating the imminent infinite. Should these simple measures fail, then the books recommended that the bed be similarly rotated, thus adjusting the overall position in relation to the Earth's magnetic field. This was an exhausting exercise, damaging to carpets, injurious to my back and provided an unnatural end for at least two elderly double beds of my acquaintance.

Overall, it seemed to me that the writers of these books had little day to day experience of ECG machines in Crigglethorpe. Even when we bought our brand new, up-to-date battery driven model (*circa* 1965), the daunting problem of 'AC' remained. I was forced to evolve my own theories and a suitable practical method of solution.

First, there was the lead. Coming from exposure to the searching, cold Yorkshire north wind into the roaring, overwhelming heat of a miner's fire, there was an obvious hazard from condensation. Cleaning the lead with a spirit-soaked rag, drying and then heating the lead became an essential preliminary ritual before the clinical could even be contemplated. Should the interference persist I was then forced to face the problem of the plugs.

Is the electric blanket still plugged in? Whether switched on or not, a plugged-in electric blanket can provide a nasty shock to even the most modern ECG machine. It leaves a layer of static that can be cut with a knife. Not only can such a layer prove detrimental to things electrical; an unwary doctor examining a patient can get a nasty shock from one lying immersed in static. It has happened to me more times than I care to remember. That is why I now always make it a rule to wear Wellington boots whenever I attend a patient with chest pain. I once wrote to the agony column of the *British Medical Journal* about this difficulty. Little came but a stream of literature from manufacturers of electric blankets.

So, I always unplug the electric blanket – and anything else in the vicinity. And I always switch off the plug sockets, in case any electrical fluid seeps out.

There have been times when even these diligent steps have proved ineffective and I have needed to switch off the whole electrical supply at the mains. This almost guarantees a perfect tracing, always supposing that you can find your way back to the bedroom and locate your ECG. You must also be prepared to cope with the inevitable trail of domestic havoc occasioned by such a dramatic manoeuvre, in the shape of ruined freezers, stopped clocks, imperfect videos and so on. Apart from the effect on the electrical impedimenta of life, it almost goes without saying that you will be deprived of light. Because of this, in my later years and more experienced, I would send the spouse down to the cellar to disconnect and reconnect the supply. Unfortunately, muffled cries in the darkness became a common complication of the procedure and, on several occasions, I have had the embarrassing experience of having to ask the ambulance, taking my official patient to coronary care, to drop off the spouse at casualty to get their leg, ankle or arm fixed.

On four occasions my routine was unsuccessful. Each time the patient was a woman in the later stages of her youth, but unaware of how late a stage. All were wearing glamorous nylon nightdresses. Now, while being aware of my own susceptibility to electricity – I have been shocked on several occasions by nylon nighties – I had no reasonable doubt that I had stumbled across a fundamental scientific fact when the 'AC

Problem' persisted in the presence of these garments, all other causes having been excluded. So, on the next occurrence of the syndrome, I ask the lady in question to remove her nightie. Her husband returned from the cellar having switched off the electricity to find his ailing wife in puris naturalibus, lit only by a single candle (I always carry one in case of power cuts). I found it difficult to explain to him the scientific nature of the exercise. Perhaps the mayonnaise smeared over her body distracted him from my explanation. I did reassure him of the health of his wife's heart, but, somehow, it did not seem to cut much ice. It is difficult to be convincing under such circumstances, especially when dressed in Wellington boots, even green ones.

Now, I may have misled you into thinking that the management of things electrical is a simple matter of logic and that the correct course of action is based on scientific principles. Unfortunately this is not so, for there are other more subtle electrical forces at work in our atmosphere. I need only mention radio waves. These became apparent during my management of what came to be known as the 'Briggs case'.

I was, in my early days, haunted by Ernest Briggs: he had more episodes of chest pain than I care to remember. He was an enigma. At 7 a.m. one morning, the telephone announced another episode in his ever-unfolding history. I was determined, as I climbed from my bed to a frosty day, that this time I would sort him out. ECG in hand, I hunted him out to his retreat in the back bedroom and with unparalleled efficiency set up the machine. There were no interference, hiccups, or abnormalities until I reached the early chest leads. Suddenly, from the machine came a voice. 'Five to eight. Time for "Lift up your Hearts".' Then solemn organ music. Exactly what happened next is a blur of tachycardia, a collapsed, whey-faced wife and the incessant ringing of ambulance bells. I hastily constructed a referral letter which sounded vaguely clinical and included my ECG tracing. This latter was a cause of considerable interest in cardiac circles for some time afterwards, especially V3, V4, V5 and V6. Perhaps a skilled musician may have been able to discern in them the musical outlines of 'O God Our Help in Ages Past'.

I do not wish to dwell unduly long on the practical aspects of electrocardiology, but there are important philosophical and behavioural aspects even in this technical area of medicine. For example, why, when you choose to reassure the most neurotic of patients with an ECG, do you inevitably find a minute but inexplicable abnormality? And why does the most classical myocardial infarction fail to produce changes in the trace? Life is simply not fair. In reviewing all the cardiographs I had done over a period of three years, I found that half of them were done for reassurance. Moreover, half of those done for reassurance concerned married couples: this interesting fact reassures me that even in today's uneasy state of marriage, it is not uncommon to find two hearts beating as one. Just occasionally, this phenomenon can go to extremes.

The couple who most typically exemplified this interesting sociological aspect of cardiology were Norma and Frank Wainwright. Frank requested a visit because Norma had been up all night with an upset stomach. There was no urgency. I called around midday, heard the story again from Frank, and went upstairs to see Norma. She was her usual bright self, but somewhat pale. She had felt cold and 'trembly' all night and had been sick a couple of times. I felt nothing untoward in her over-large tummy and I started to chat about gastric flu and related topics. My hand naturally strayed to her pulse, which registered little. As I was writing the prescription for a stomach-soothing mixture, it occurred to me that I had actually been unable to feel any pulsation at all at her wrist. I tried again. There was the merest flutter. I listened to her heart and could barely count the rate. The ECG recorded a ventricular tachycardia of about 200 plus. I gave her IV lignocaine – a risky business, but it was all the rage then – and arranged her transfer to the local coronary care unit, where she was successfully cardioverted.

Thelma, their daughter, phoned the following morning to ask if I would call to see her father, since he was most upset and shocked by the previous day's drama. He was sitting by the fire, agitated. 'That hospital drive nearly finished me', he said, 'I could hardly breathe, when I got in.' I felt his pulse. It was rapid and totally irregular. He admitted his chest had been tight. An ECG confirmed a myocardial infarction with atrial fibrillation. I asked the SHO about the availability of double beds in the unit, but he did not seem particularly amused; in fact, I do not think he believed me. I visited them that evening. They were lying side by side in single beds, discussing the day's events. Apart from the wiring and the somewhat repetitive pictures on their individual televisions, they might have been in their own bedroom in Jubilee Street.

Yet, even the most technical aspect of medicine must, eventually, be applied to the individual and it is in this application that the exact is blurred to the empirical and the science of medicine becomes an art. Life does not begin or end with an ECG recording – well, not often, anyway. Not uncommonly, the ECG is the beginning of what is now called an 'ongoing situation'. The handling of such a situation requires tact, understanding and not a little nous. Some people would say it might also require a degree of counselling skill. Personally, I am even less adept at counselling than I am at managing machinery; I did try the art once but failed. Generally speaking, I have now resorted to 'telling'.

The story of Fred and Vera Brook epitomises for me the sheer helplessness of machinery when faced with the biology and psychology of the living human being – especially when I have chosen to facilitate the interaction with my own brand of counselling. It began simply enough. Fred came to see me and gave a typical history of angina. We discussed the implications and I was able to demonstrate some ischaemic changes on the ECG. He wished to continue working as a senior clerk for the NCB. His main stress, he admitted, was the hassle of getting to work, what with the traffic and everything. I suggested that he might travel a few minutes earlier and return a few minutes later, and I still do not consider this to be extravagant advice. As he was leaving, he asked if I would take care not to reveal his condition to his wife, for she worried unduly. A week or two later, Vera came to see me and, as was her wont, burst into tears as soon as she sat down. 'It's me husband', she wept, 'He's got another woman. He goes to work much earlier than before and he's always home late'. I suggested that there may be other reasons and that few love affairs, in my experience, flourished only from 8 a.m. to 8. 30 a.m. and from 5 p.m. to 5.30 p.m. She was not consoled. 'But why should he suddenly change his habits?' she asked. My Hippocratic Oath prevented me from revealing the truth. When Frank returned for follow-up, I suggested that it might be as well if he put her in the picture. There was no chance. What about doing something to ease her loneliness? I felt sure that this was the root of her chronic unhappiness. Perhaps a dog might help – I had read of the value of pets in rehabilitation: I had in mind a cosy Yorkie or Peke. He would think about it.

Some days later, while out on my visits, I was struck by the sight of a middle-aged lady travelling at admirable speed up the steep hill of Cliff Road. As I passed I realised that she was being pulled by a fearsome pair of young English Setters; she tried to wave, but could not. Her smile was not, in fact, a smile, but rather the fixed grimace of the trapped. Later that week, both the setters appeared in the 'Pets' section of the Small Ads in the local press. Fred told me she had phoned the newspaper from the ward as soon as she got over the fixing of her fractured tibia. He further told me that he had decided to take early retirement on medical grounds, so that he could look after her. 'It suits me as well', he said.

My relationship with my ECG machine has been forged over the years in the twin fires of expectation and disappointment but has now settled to a wary companionship born of reality. The machine itself no longer has the shining cover of its youth and the corners are scuffed and worn. The hinges are rusting and cracked and the lid must be opened gently. It runs down more easily than before and consumes batteries faster than I remember. Sometimes, if the wind is cold or the humidity is high, it produces a curiously wavy trace. There are even days when it will not work at all. I sense that it does not take kindly to the authoritarian approach of the practice nurse: it needs cossetting a little to produce a good performance and, above all, it needs time.

We have grown together, me and my ECG machine.

RONALD MULROY

Wakefield

3
Cardiac Arrest

No emergency in medicine is more dramatic than a cardiac arrest, and its management is truly a matter of life or death. Successful treatment depends upon prompt and efficient action but even in hospital, where trained staff and appropriate equipment are immediately available, management is often a matter of barely organised chaos. When arrest occurs out of hospital the dice are loaded against the doctor or the lay resuscitator and a successful outcome is all the more rewarding.

Arrested Development

One Spring afternoon, after a gruelling shift as a Casualty SHO I discovered that a doctor is never off duty. I had relinquished my white coat and was savouring a sensation of anonymity and irresponsibility wandering around the local town's shops, when quite suddenly my aimless, fluid thoughts froze. There was a curious tension in the air, emanating from a huddle of people nearby. My mind made one decision but my legs another and I found myself ambling, then hurrying, towards the throng. At its epicentre was a moribund individual: unconscious, blue and, clearly, pulseless. The clouds parted and a celestial finger jabbed me in the chest. 'OK,' He said. 'You're it.' My moment had come.

'I am a doctor', I heard someone say with startling authority and clarity. It was me. Expectant eyes turned towards me and then back to the Arrested One. Already, 'ABC, Airway/Breathing/Circulation' was echoing, mantra-like, in my brain and I knelt into action. Loosen collar, clear airway, extend neck . . . I slid automatically into the familiar resuscitation routine. Working feverishly, I suppressed pangs of panic as I realised that I would be without the comfort of the cardiac arrest team bustling to my assistance. But He who had poked me in the chest came to the rescue, dragging a startled local GP, festooned with carrier bags, from a nearby supermarket. Without a word he adopted the role of oxygenator; he blew, I pumped. After a while, I blew and he pumped. Then I grinned and he paused. I had noticed some of his shopping, which had spilled from its bag onto the pavement: double cream, butter and a packet of cigarettes. Sheepishly, he redoubled his efforts. The faint sound of an ambulance siren was just audible; meanwhile, the audience gawped.

And then I noticed a strange phenomenon. While, supposedly, a whole life flashes before the eyes of the dying, I now realise that rather bizarre memories leap simultaneously into the mind of the resuscitator – particularly in the disorientating environment of a shopping mall, without the reassuring blur of bleeps, drugs, urgent voices and tangles of wire.

What I saw, as I continued the resuscitation in a curiously detached way, was a re-run of all the cardiac arrests I have ever experienced, a cardiac compilation. This must have taken only a few seconds, yet it encompassed my entire medical career. And one common thread ran through the sweat, panic, exhaustion and emotion of each: amusement.

As a medical student, the simple duty of holding a cardiac arrest bleep was sufficient to render me mute with terror. My ultimate nightmare was to be first on the scene before the arrest team. As a result, I deliberately spent a great deal of time tripping over, tying my shoelaces or going to the bank en route to cardiac arrests. In urgent situations, when I happened to be uncomfortably close to the danger zone, I would simply run away, although I lived in fear of colliding with the crash team which would be hurtling along in the opposite direction. The easiest option was, of course, to secrete myself in the nearest toilet. In this way I discovered that fear is not necessarily overcome by status for once, when I arrived breathlessly in my hiding place, I discovered the duty houseman there too. We exchanged embarrassed and guilty looks, then ran dutifully to the ward, each trying to be just slightly slower than the other. Legend has it that inexperienced medical registrars and anaesthetists have similarly sought sanctuary under the pretext of answering the call of nature. Presumably, the nursing staff soon adapt to this system by simply wheeling the arrested patient along to the nearest toilet.

My metamorphosis into a houseman brought a confidence built around a few successful resuscitations. All junior doctors know that such a state of equilibrium is inevitably transient: medical banana-skins lie just around the corner. And so it was that, one day and for no obvious reason, my few skills deserted me at the scene of an arrest. I was unable to intubate, insert a drip or do anything other than gibber. Perhaps in sympathy, the ECG ran out of paper so another was fetched hurriedly. As the machine hummed and the paper ran, it printed an ominously featureless line: asystole. The members of the team regarded each other knowingly. My composure by this time regained I gave a sigh, a wise head on very young shoulders; I was about to proclaim, solemnly, that further efforts would be futile, that we should withdraw gracefully, when someone pointed out that the second ECG had not actually been connected to the patient. The various members of the team emitted noises of incredulity and pointed fingers of blame at each other. Rapidly the situation was resolved and, at last, I was poised with defibrillation paddles. 'Stand back' I said in what would have been a commanding voice had it not been a dry throated, nervous squeak. To my horror, as the patient jerked so too did the anaesthetist. And having jerked, he convulsed and frothed, muscles twitching and eyes rolling, his audience aghast. Then he smiled – his little joke.

Most cardiac arrests were less traumatic – for myself if not the patient. Some were downright bizarre. One particular medical registrar with a reputation for flamboyance, and what might be charitably described as an offbeat sense of humour, was fond of transforming resuscitations into game shows.

Registrar (faced by patient refractory, thus far, to his efforts): 'OK, who has never given an intracardiac injection?'

The audience's gaze falls on me.

Registrar: 'Dr H, come on down!'

The audience whoops and hollers in excitement then a hush falls as, trembling, I take the syringe.

Registrar: 'Now, what's the dose?'

Dr H (faltering): 'Er . . . 1 ml.'

Audience (screaming encouragement): 'Higher!'
Dr H: '5 ml?'
Audience: 'Higher, higher!'
Dr H: '10 ml?'
Registrar (to cheers of audience): 'Yeeeeeees! On you go.'
I feel for the bony landmarks and insert the needle; all is
silent and as rivulets of sweat trickle down the back, I realise
that my month-old white coat is smelling none too savoury.
My nasal contortion bestows on me a look of immense con-
centration. I slowly withdraw the plunger – blood.
Registrar: 'One hundred and eeeeeeeeighty!'
The audience erupts.
Astoundingly, the patient survived.
The sound of the ambulance siren distantly impinged upon
my consciousness. I found myself drifting back towards reality, but one cardiac event flashed into my mind before the
mental video clicked to a halt. Only a few days previously, a
middle-aged man had been brought into casualty with crush-
ing central chest pain. During the initial assessment in the
emergency room, he arrested. On this occasion, the process
went smoothly and he convulsed back into life with one shock
from the defibrillation paddles. We congratulated ourselves
and I left the scene for the medical team to arrange admission.
My swollen sensation of achievement was rudely punctured
shortly afterwards by the medical registrar, whom I met in the
coffee room. 'Do you know what his first words were when he
came round?' asked my colleague, with evident disgust, in reference to our mutual patient. 'Can I go private?' He snorted.
'And we resuscitated the bugger under the NHS.'
Back in the shopping precinct, I found myself pressing
rhythmically on an unknown person's chest. Noting that he
was beginning to look distinctly pink, I felt for a pulse. Miracle
of miracles. A strong, regular beat. I experienced various
sensations at this point, all of which require tired clichés to provide adequate description. My heart missed a beat, I felt tingl-
ing up and down my spine, that sort of thing. The sum total
was that I felt both delighted and amazed. 'Grrrmphthnrg'
said my previously fibrillating friend. 'Frrthmphtnth'. This, of
course, was music to my ears. The Heavenly Hand gave a

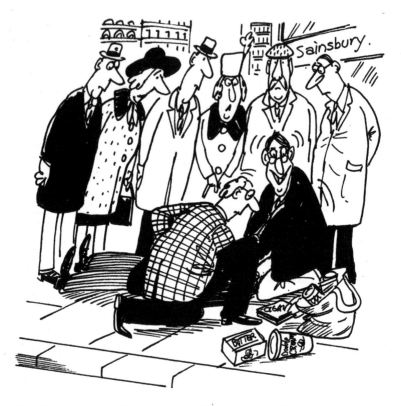

I had just noticed some of his shopping . . . double cream, butter and a packet of cigarettes.

thumbs-up sign and I turned to the crowd of watching faces, expecting to see them, on cue, smiling lovingly, in soft focus. No. They continued to look gormless. One was eating fish and chips from a newspaper and seemed on the verge of offering some to the patient.

'The ambulancemen are just coming', said a voice from behind me. I turned. 'I'm a social worker', she said. 'Can I be of any assistance?'

'My God', I thought. 'Hospital doctor, GP and social worker. Let's have a case conference.'

'No thanks,' I replied, grinning sweetly and heroically through my sweat. 'He seems pretty stable now'. Before I could engage her in polite conversation regarding potential benefits to which my patient might suddenly have become entitled, it was all over. I plummeted from starring role to extra as the ambulancemen assumed control and, with nonchalant efficiency, scooped the patient onto a stretcher and into the ambulance. My hands felt conspicuously idle, oversized for my body. As the ambulance sped away, the crowd gradually dispersed and I thanked my GP colleague for his help. For a few moments I stood at the spot of the drama, now transformed effortlessly into just another few drab and faceless square yards of shopping precinct. I felt quite odd. No cardiac arrest had ever affected me before: white coats and clinical setting provide armour-like protection for the emotions. Or perhaps the amusement just-recalled so vividly that I have always derived from resuscitation is a subconscious mechanism designed to displace more profound or uncomfortable sensations. Now, having dealt with a cardiac arrest outside the hospital setting, out of context, I felt . . . emotional.

I pondered this. Maybe it was the unexpected success, or being poked in the chest by God; maybe I was simply tired. But I sensed that I was on the verge of some discovery or fulfilment, some breathtaking spiritual enlightenment. I loitered around for a few minutes awaiting an apparition, a bolt from the blue or some meaningful symbol. A child walked by, picking his nose. After that, nothing else happened.

That evening I lay on my bed, trying to relax in an effort to suppress an inexplicable tachycardia. I considered the heart. Lucky old heart. Guts gurgle, nerves twang, lungs wheeze, rattle and roll but, in the orchestra of anatomy, the heart sings. The metronome of passion, it may race, pound or miss a beat. It is a badge of attributes, an emblem of the generous (kind hearted), brave (lion hearted) or friendly (warm hearted). Hearts reflect the capriciousness of love and in so doing may ache, be broken or be lost completely. So popular an organ is it that no one has the heart to insult it: hence a dodgy ticker rather than a bad heart. But my heart felt strange. Empty and sad . . . heavy. That was it. I felt heavy hearted. So heavy, in fact, that I was dragging my heart on a lead ten yards behind me. All this because of an unresolved incident in a shopping centre, an incident which I felt sure had been designed to be meaningful.

In search of inspiration, I looked up 'heart' in my dictionary. The fact that the preceding entry was 'hearse' did not escape my notice. 'Heart: 1a. A hollow muscular organ that by its rhythmic contraction acts as a force pump maintaining the circulation of the blood'. This I knew already. '1b. The breast, bosom'. I skipped a few lines until I reached 3a: 'Humane disposition; compassion. 3b. Love, affection. 3c. Courage, spirit'. This seemed more hopeful. '4. One's innermost character or feelings'. I felt that the truth was within my grasp; impatiently, I turned the page. '5. The central or innermost part of a cabbage, lettuce, etc.' I groaned. The next entry was, appropriately, heartache, 'mental anguish, sorrow'. Wearily, I scanned the nearby columns. Heartbeat . . . heartfelt . . . heart to heart . . . I stopped. Heart to heart. That was it. 'Frank or intimate talk'. I slammed the dictionary shut. My eyes narrowed and my tachycardia increased. I knew what I had to do.

The voice on the telephone was full of mock admiration. 'So you're the little hero who resuscitated him in the street.' I made embarrassed noises. Sister on duty in the coronary care unit was a friend of mine; it seemed there would be no problem. 'I know it's outside of visiting hours but I'd like to talk to him. Just for a few minutes.' 'Well, he's perfectly stable, sitting up in bed and chatting. Come over when you like. I'm sure he'd like to pat his lifesaver on the back.' My protests that my mind was on weightier matters than mere congratulations were met by the click of the receiver as she put the phone down. For a few minutes I sat, staring into space, rehearsing an imaginary conversation. Then with an air of resolution I left my room, crossed the road, entered the hospital and went along to the coronary care unit.

Sister was on the telephone; she gestured towards Bed 3. There he was. Sitting up, conscious, pink and with a regular pulse. A monitor by his bedside blipped reassuringly. He looked thoughtful and this pleased me. Diffidently, I introduced myself as someone who had been there 'when it happened' and he seemed to understand immediately who I was and what I had done for him. This I interpreted as Sister having forewarned him of my visit rather than divine intervention. He thanked me profusely and we had an awkward, stilted conversation. Stupidly, I asked him how he felt. 'Fine,' he replied, 'apart from these bruised ribs.' I smiled, embarrassed and apologetic. Our conversation meandered harmlessly up a number of cul-de-sacs and after a few minutes I rose to leave, mumbling platitudes. The Heavenly Hand shoved me back in my chair; the time had come. I cleared my throat as if to swallow the previous irrelevant conversation. 'There is one thing I'd like to ask. . . .' I began, uncertainly. 'I hope you won't mind.' He looked interested. 'When you were . . . you know . . .' 'Nearly dead?' he asked. I nodded, relieved at his understanding. 'What did you feel? Did you see or hear anything? Did you experience anything, a journey . . . or . . . or . . .' My inquiry tapered off into vague questioning gestures. My vocabulary was inadequate to express the enormity of the question I was asking.

For a very long time he frowned, considering, remembering. I envisaged choirs of angels, symbolic bridges, tunnels leading to enlightenment. In my mind, heavenly music reached a crescendo. He spoke. 'No.' I looked startled; he too seemed taken aback. 'No, nothing, I'm afraid. I don't remember anything about it.' 'Ah well,' I said. My smile masked my disappointment. 'I just, you know, wondered.'

As I stood, he spoke again, an effort of memory on his face. 'There was one thing . . .' I froze. 'It sounds so ridiculous that I'm almost too embarrassed to mention it.' My knuckles whitened as my hand gripped the chair. 'I remember . . .' 'Yes?' I gasped, 'go on.' 'I remember . . . a smell.' He brightened as the memory returned in full. 'A smell of fish and chips.' I turned and left.

And that was it. No revelation, no real ending. Just the knowledge that, when the Grim Reaper finally calls, you might get a whiff of whatever's been frying locally, if you are lucky. As I trudged out of the coronary care unit, though my heart did not necessarily sing, I felt instantly better.

KEITH HOPCROFT

Basildon

Perks of the Job

Having walked for five years in hallowed halls, at first as a junior minion, then as a senior minion, treading softly in the footsteps of worthy masters – cardiologists, rheumatologists, chest physicians, general physicians with an Interest, others with less interest and one with a blinding passion, though not in medicine. Patrick Martin, single, 33 years of age and a late developer, looked up one night and saw a great flash of light in the sky. And when it had gone he heard a voice crying:

'Renounce the ways of the wards, Patrick. Cast off your white coat, put aside your Hospital Medicine diary with tables of normal values and tests of adrenal function, throw away all those grubby little bits of paper, torch pens and boiled sweets which fill up your white coat pockets, and put on your tweed jacket and brogues.'

Patrick did all these things as the Oracle commanded, handed in his bleep and kissed the switchboard operator, and was born again that day as a country GP.

In fact he had been on the lookout for the Oracle recently. The esoteric world of general medicine, with or without an interest, had attracted him since his student days and six months as a house physician in a busy provincial hospital convinced him that this was the most exciting discovery since they found that bread could not only be sliced but toasted in front of an open fire and covered with fresh dairy butter and home-made marmalade.

The job was short on supervision and long on happenings. He thought on his feet as routine, often ate on them and occasionally slept on them. They were fast becoming the most valuable parts of his anatomy. On his first night on call he was summoned to a desperately ill man who was cold, sweating and choking and quite unable to speak. At his teaching hospital Patrick had seen many patients with motor neurone disease but had to recall his textbooks and lectures to diagnose acute pulmonary oedema, and had never heard this awful death rattle before. He switched on the oxygen and injected him with the potion he had learned. Next morning the patient was sitting up in bed, breathing quietly and drinking tea when Patrick began his ward round, and neither of them ever forgot that experience. At the end of six months of treating countless similar emergencies, often successfully and usually single-handed, Patrick felt that walking on water was no big problem. Patients and nurses vied in their admiration for him and ward clerks lowered their heads when addressing him.

However, after another year spent displaying his magical powers in teaching and postgraduate hospitals throughout the great metropolis to rather less appreciative audiences, it was clearly time to become a registrar. This gave him greater status: he was allowed to put his hands in is pockets on ward rounds, but he discovered to his dismay that it was much less fun. It was also quite hazardous. Not only did he see the patients that the houseman had not already three-quarters cured, he also had to think of something intelligent to say to the consultant that neither houseman nor consultant had thought of first. As he became more skilled at this new exercise of hospital medicine gamesmanship Patrick began to realise that the consultant's role could be quite severely undermined by a competent team of juniors, unless he super-specialised by developing a skill in inserting fibre-optic instruments into cavities where no instrument had gone before. This did not appeal to him, as his great enjoyment of general medicine was in its infinite variety.

It was at about this time that he underwent a slow metamorphosis. He found he was spending rather a lot of time talking to the patients. Not 'Have your bowel actions always been green and slimy?' talking; more 'How do you stop the slugs eating your lupins, then?'. He found that many patients were interesting people and in fact they were frequently more interesting than their illnesses. He tried to keep this sacrilegious discovery to himself for fear of being pushed sideways into psychiatry, where they had nothing better to do than talk to people all day. It was only when he tried to explain to his boss how this communication business was becoming more important to him, and how he felt he might be heading in the wrong direction by extending his understanding of anal sphincter pressures by going on a course, that his boss gave him that 'I

must have been wrong about you all along' look and said in
farewell, 'Well, the best of luck, old chap, but I'm afraid you'll
be wasted in general practice.'

If being a hospital doctor was all about seeing, investigating
and discussing people with rare diseases, which Patrick did
not believe it was, then the boss was right. In his first 15 years
in general practice he did not see a single case of Syringomyelia,
Duchenne dystrophy or Charcot-Marie-Tooth disease. If he
did see them he misdiagnosed them as virus infections, but
then, if he had managed to spot a case, he would not have been
able to cure it or find another doctor who could. In fact, if
Patrick had sat down at the end of fifteen years and made a list
of those conditions he had not seen since leaving hospital it
would have been as long as his arm, and his other arm, both
legs and three times around his waist.

It came as a severe shock at first to discover that the vast
majority of patients he saw with chest pain had not suffered a
heart attack, or a spontaneous pneumothorax, or a pulmonary
embolus, or in fact any of the other seventeen causes of chest
pain that he had learned to pass his higher examinations, and
which seemed to adequately cover most of the patients he used
to see in hospital with that symptom. He began to wonder who
managed to find these unfortunate souls with serious but quite
interesting conditions that he was clearly missing, but who
found their way into the medical wards. Most of Patrick's
patients left the surgery with a label of '?muscular pain' and a
combined diagnosis and prognosis of 'I don't know what it is
but I'm sure it isn't serious', which did not always reassure the
sufferer as much as Patrick hoped it would. He was not yet experienced enough to tell patients they were suffering from
fibrositis or rheumatism, having not yet discovered that these
conditions might exist; a pity, because as he later learned many
people found these terms reassuring since it was a great relief
to hear they had not had heart attacks.

Patrick recalled that some of his more brilliant diagnoses as
a house physician were made with a deal of luck and a peer
into the retrospectoscope. He remembered one middle-aged
lady being brought into the emergency room in a coma, with
no previous medical history and very few helpful physical

signs except a flattish nervous system and a flatter blood pressure. The great doctor scratched his head, took some blood for posterity, resolving to fill in the biochemistry request form when some intelligent thoughts filled his head, and put up a dextrose–saline drip. After a few minutes the patient woke up and Patrick realised he had accidently cured an Addisonian Crisis. Working backwards he wrote 'plasma cortisol' on the empty form and stood back to receive the tumultuous applause.

Three months into general practice Patrick visited a frail old lady in her late seventies who had been feeling 'all faint and weak' for some time, and who was hypotensive. He wondered if she might have a 'silent' coronary, and did an electrocardiogram. It did not confirm his suspicions but he remembered the last odd case of low blood pressure he had seen, and he had her plasma cortisol measured. It was barely recordable and she was rejuvenated with cortisone supplements. For years to come after that he checked the plasma cortisol on every person with low blood pressure but never found another case in the rest of his career.

After six months of seeing people who did not yet have fibrositis or rheumatism Patrick broke his luck. Alfred Morris, a thirty-six-year-old postman, had a very severe pain in the middle of his chest and even his Auntie Maureen could have told him it was a heart attack. Patrick did an ECG and sent it in with the accompanying letter to the houseman (just in case they did not have an electrocardiograph in the hospital) explaining (lest the entire medical team had never seen one before) that it showed an anterior infarction. Mr Morris came home ten days later having had a few minor twinges but otherwise making a good recovery. A couple of days later Patrick made a routine visit to offer his advice on becoming ambulant again.

'I'm glad you've come, doctor', said Mrs Morris at the door. 'He doesn't feel too well.' Alfred Morris did not look too well either. His skin had a rather ominous waxy appearance but he greeted the doctor cheerily enough, so Patrick thought he could not be too bad. 'I keep coming over swimy, doc.'

His wife helped to peel off several layers of winter clothing and Patrick slid a stethoscope over Alfred's chest, hovering for some time over the area where he usually managed to find the heart. The doctor turned a shade paler than the patient at this point, no mean feat as Mr Morris's face was rapidly graduating through some of the more virginal degrees of whiteness. Patrick could hear the *lubs* and *dups* which told him that the heart was still going through the motions, but he only managed to count twenty a minute and they were fading fast. 'Let's check the old blood pressure', he said in what was intended to be a breezy sort of voice. He eventually succeeded in tracking it down. The top bit was around 50 and the bottom bit about 45. Patrick mused that this was not a level that he would have thought compatible with continuing to sit in a chair and wondered when he would fall off. He pulled himself together, abandoned the breezy sort of voice and decided on a calm, measured explanation of the situation as he saw it. 'Wegottogetyouintohospital', he explained calmly. 'Ok doc, you know best. Can I go to the loo first? I've just had my water tablet.'

He stood up before Patrick had time to scream 'No!' and took one step towards the door. He swivelled back and started to form an expression that was probably going to be a silly grin, but which disappeared in the middle like the Cheshire Cat's. Then at last he fell over.

Patrick speculated on how he would cope with a cardiac arrest in the absence of a defibrillator, a drip set, an endotracheal tube or any of those terribly useful aids one found in hospital – in particular, large numbers of other doctors and a plentiful supply of nurses handing apparatus and syringes of life-restorer. His speculation was interrupted by a noise from the unusually immobile patient. It was one of those incredibly deep sighs people make after a cardiac arrest, and which is not normally followed by any further respiratory activity. A rapid and limited assessment of Alfred Morris's prone frame satisfied him that no further activity was to be anticipated in any other system unless he thought of something very clever and very soon.

A distant bell tinkled. When Patrick was a fledgling houseman an anaesthetist asked his tutorial group, 'What is the first thing you do with a patient who has arrested?' Rejecting suggestions of cardiac massage, lung massage, injections of adrenaline, calcium and the application of various tubes and pipes, he shouted, 'Rubbish! You give him an almighty thump on the chest,' and demonstrated the process with his fist on the desk, causing a decanter of water, his notes and the lectern to leap six inches in to the air.

So that is what Patrick did.

He failed to induce any acts of levitation but something even more remarkable happened. Alfred's heart started beating. Nothing extravagant – about once every five seconds at first. Followed by a breath. Then another. Then the whole biological orchestra struck up. The heart moved into a gentle andante at a rate of sixty or so, the lungs instinctively remembered what they had been taught by the nurses in hospital and began to inflate and deflate at twenty breaths a minute, then the central nervous system caught on and the head went into a cadenza. The eyes opened, and the silly grin finished where it had frozen a short lifetime ago. Finally the mouth opened. Here was the moment of truth. Patrick held his breath expectantly. Would he perhaps speak in tongues, or deliver a cryptic but deeply meaningful account of the hereafter?

'Bugger me', revealed the born-again agnostic, and rubbed his chest. Giving his wife strict instructions not to let him anywhere near the toilet he rushed to the phone, and within a few minutes they were all in the coronary ambulance. After great clanging of bells Alfred found himself back in the coronary care unit without further excitement. The houseman gave Patrick an oddly incredulous look when he explained why he had not had time to write an admission letter this time. The GP shrugged and went off to have a cup of tea.

Mr Morris came home three days later. Patrick equipped himself with an airway and a prayer mat and revisited his patient. Mr Morris met him at the door this time, and Patrick ushered him in before something awful happened. 'No need to worry, doc. I'm a lot better today. Sorry I made such a fuss last time you came. They told me all about it on the ward.' 'What did they tell you?' Patrick wondered whether they were wise to tell Alfred the whole truth. But he need not have worried. 'They said it was a fainting attack. Low blood pressure, apparently. Water tablets too strong.'

He nodded reassuringly. Not a bad story. 'I'm not so sure though. Look at this, doc'. He undid his shirt and showed the doctor a bruise over his sternum. 'Now I don't know how that happened but it don't half hurt. There was a bloke in my ward who had a really bad turn. The doctor jumped up and down on his chest – you could see him through the curtains – and he was pretty sore when he woke up. But nothing like that happened to me, I'd have noticed it, wouldn't I?' Patrick agreed that it was rather odd, but suggested it would settle down in the next week or so. Having satisfied himself that normal service had been resumed in the Morris household, he prepared to leave.

'Just a minute, doc', said the flourishing postman, and produced a camera. 'I know you've been very good to me and I'd like to have a little memento. Would you mind if my wife took a picture of us together?' Glowing with pride Patrick agreed, and they posed outrageously with his stethoscope on the patient's chest, smiling at the camera with Alfred looking up at him like an adoring dog while Mrs Morris pressed the button.

'I like to do my own printing, so I'll show you the result next time you come doc.'

A couple of days later Mr Morris's discharge summary arrived in the surgery, signed by the medical registrar. It informed the GP that the ECG on admission showed no change and that the diagnosis of this admission was 'syncopal attack'. It seemed that they really believed their own fairy story.

It was less than a year since Patrick Martin had worked in hospital and not too many years since he was a medical student. He recalled teaching hospital consultants waving scraps of paper allegedly from GPs, asking him to 'Please see and treat.' He recalled even more clearly the condescension displayed by housemen (less sensitive than he) who had doubtless been shown the same letter in their formative years, to some GPs (who could not even be bothered to write an admission note at all) and rued the contempt with which doctors could dismiss events described by others – whether patients or other doctors – which they had not witnessed themselves. Patrick reflected that he did not save lives very often in general practice, and certainly not in such a dramatic and unequivocal manner, so on this rare occasion he controlled his outrage with some difficulty when informed officially that his patient had merely fainted. Even the patient seemed to know better than that.

Patrick looked forward to his next visit to the postman. Alfred was now out of any danger and he regarded the call as partly a social event and also as a sort of presentation ceremony. On only one previous occasion had he been given a present by a patient. Actually it was the widow of the patient, an uncomplaining man whose stomach cancer Patrick had missed until it was too late. Perhaps it was always too late, but Patrick was remorseful and devoted much time to helping the couple cope with the last few weeks. For all this he received a gift of a silver pillbox, probably the most precious item the old man possessed, but which his sad, bereft widow insisted he would have wanted his doctor to have.

This would be a lighter occasion, though. Having confirmed that Alfred's clinical improvement was being maintained, he went to the window where Alfred produced from a large brown paper bag a carefully produced black-and-white print depicting the happy pair.

'There you are, doc. You can have it as it is with my compliments.' He paused, and it was clear that an even better offer was to come. 'If you really like it, I can put it in a nice frame for you for a fiver.' Patrick Martin had it framed, and kept it on his mantelpiece next to the pillbox so that he would always remember how rewarding general practice could be.

P.J. SOUTH

Frittenden

Mary, Mary

Mary had a cigarette
In paper white as snow,
And everywhere that Mary went
She'd pant and puff and blow

'What makes poor Mary stagger so,
And look like she might die?'
'She's had a heart attack, you know',
The doctor did reply

MARIE CAMPKIN
London

Humpty Dumpty

Humpty Dumpty sat on a wall,
Wouldn't go out walking at all,
Serum cholesterol mounted and then –
Humpty: RIP. Amen

MARIE CAMPKIN
London

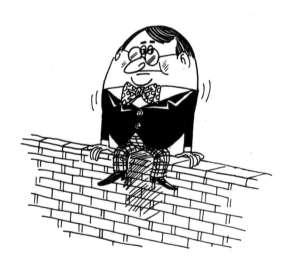

4
Recollections

Some of the contributors to this anthology are unashamedly autobio-graphical. The authors unlock their memories to produce conversational recollections of things that happened when they were students or junior doctors, or even children, and which have something to do with hearts.

An Education of Hearts

I had an early education about hearts from my father. He had a maxim.

A conscientious and kindly old-style GP he looked after 6000 demanding, urban patients single-handedly during the war. He worked incredibly hard, holding three surgeries on most days and doing as many as thirty visits; I knew about these marathon rounds as I used to count the names and addresses when I was allowed to help write out the visiting list. At least petrol rationing ensured that there were no traffic problems in those days, but the car was carefully driven as it had to last out the war.

Besides attending to the surgeries and calls he operated at the cottage hospital, was medical officer to the local aircraft factory and spent sleepless nights on ARP duty. This, he said, was the most wearying task of all not because of the loss of sleep, but because of the behaviour of the ladies in the ARP centre; he developed a side effect from these nights which lasted ever after; he could not stand anyone knitting by the fireside. Every time a bomb fell the ladies in the ARP post would all stop knitting as though a conductor had waved his baton at them. My father compared them to the old hags who sat waiting for the guillotine to do its ghastly work in the French Revolution. After the bomb had exploded they would unanimously wag their heads; I do not think they actually cackled but they might as well have from the effect they had on him; and they resumed their knitting – click click click – until the next bomb.

He survived his war by organisation and forethought and refused to wear himself out. 'Never run,' he said, 'except to haemorrhages and fires. Collect yourself for heart attacks.' I do not know what he would have made of the galloping cardiac arrest teams of today that thunder, bleeps and bells resounding, along hospital corridors while other patients crouch round-eyed, and no doubt palpitating, beneath their bed-clothes. How many more heart attacks do they cause?

My father's remark was usually provoked by being summoned urgently to a case of 'collapse'. 'Collapse', he reckoned, usually meant that the patient would either be dead by the time he arrived, in which case to rush in panting, red and sweaty-faced was unseemly, or else he or she would be found 'digging for Victory' in their cabbage patch. They had perhaps felt a little faint during their unaccustomed exertion in the hot afternoon sun. It was ten to one that they would already have been cured by a solicitous neighbour and a cup of hot, sweet tea.

A third possibility was the 'Family Row Collapse'. Good old-fashioned family rows were known to be potent provokers of strokes and heart attacks. A stately entrance here by the urgently summoned doctor could be more definitely efficacious. Silence would fall among the opposing factions and the heat would suddenly cool. 'Collect yourself before you arrive', said my father, 'You will be more useful when you get there and it will save you and all of them from having coronaries.'

For haemorrhages, however, my father moved fast. Often they were the result of obstetric emergencies. At five or six years old I was not meant to know what an obstetric emergency was, but not much escapes the beady eye and sharp ears of doctors' children when the practice is in the house, especially when the children occasionally indulge in a little un-vetted telephone answering. This was a gripping occupation as far as I was concerned. I puffed up with importance as I lifted the receiver and used my most grown-up answering voice. I usually only got my hands on the phone when my mother was out as my telephone reception duties were certainly not officially encouraged, but Maud, the maid, connived. Poor Maud weighed fifteen stone and liked to put her feet up whenever my mother's back was turned, but she was the best that could be found in war-time and since she was only too happy to let me run to the telephone if it disturbed her repose I adored her.

Having answered, I would write down careful messages containing the name, the address and the 'Problem'. Important messages such as 'heart attacks' and even 'found dead' were splendid; sore throats and the like were more run of the mill. I learned, in a Pavlovian way, to equate the various messages with different evoked responses. The mention of a haemorrhage, especially if coming from a midwife, led to instantaneous drama. The maid would waddle off rapidly to search out my father, usually to be found in quiet moments in the dispensary making up lovely bottles of red medicine, wrapping them in stiff white paper and sealing them with red sealing wax, or he would be pounding away with his mortar and pestle – very relaxing.

Within moments the car, protected (against bomb fragments) by two mattresses on the roof would roar down the road and (on its return) there would be oblique but fascinating enquiries from my mother. 'Did you have to use the forceps, dear?' Since the only forceps I knew about were those used for tweezing splinters out of fingers I found it difficult to understand all the excitement.

Heart attacks evoked a quieter response. The medical bag would be checked first for morphine. The exit from the house was speedy but more considered. You could almost see the words of reassurance to anxious relatives forming on my father's lips ready to issue forth as soon as he arrived. I soon learned that these visits might take a long time, as one of my treats was to join him in the car and sit outside a 'visit' until he re-emerged; I often finished reading almost a whole book. The patients rarely went to hospital. Only occasionally was my wait in the car enlivened by the clang of ambulance bells: the patients either did very well or died in their own homes. If the latter occurred a mournful but guarded account would be given to my mother when my father arrived home. Summarised, it was usually, 'Old so and so didn't make it.' A thousand words could not have been more graphic. Much better to hear was the casual, 'Oh, we pulled him through.' What and where was pulled, I wondered?

Inevitably I assimilated an important fact at a tender age. Hearts could stop. This was a great worry to me, because it seemed that I really was not meant to know exactly what was going on, and had been told on one occasion, 'You don't need to worry about that sort of thing yet!' I didn't like to ask what circumstances could cause this fearsome stoppage. Perhaps hearts just stopped. Perhaps my heart would suddenly stop. I brooded on this, especially at night, and felt real fear as I was caged into the Anderson shelter on the floor of the dining room; not the most relaxing environment for sleep, but it was not the bombs that worried me. Clasping myself to keep warm in those uncentrally heated days, by chance, I found my heartbeat.

Thereafter, I would deliberately lie with my hand on it as a safety precaution so that I would know immediately if my heart stopped and I was dead. I reasoned that if I called out urgently for help the instant that this dire event happened, my father would come and revive me as surely as he had 'pulled other people through' when we had driven out to 'heart attacks'. Thus, unconsciously, I doubted his maxim. He should run fast to my heart attack.

Eventually, however, I would drift into sleep, slumber through goodness knows how many wailings of air-raid sirens and wake in the morning to find, joy of joys, my heart still beating.

Despite these worries and somewhat to my surprise I survived my childhood. Other distractions took over, removing hearts from my broodings for a good many years, and when they reappeared in my consciousness they had become interesting subjects for pretty diagrams in red and blue. Their potential for stopping and the mechanics of keeping them going were not taken too seriously for a while. As a medical student, however, their importance re-emerged. Now they were associated with stethoscopes and were status symbols indeed. This was especially so at St Elsewhere's where, through some quirk of custom, medical students were denied the privilege of wearing white coats. The dental students wore short white coats. The housemen, registrars and more academic consultants wore long white coats. (The other breed of consultant was found in immaculate pinstripe, often with a rose in the buttonhole.) The nurses were delightful in caps, ribbons and aprons with waist-clinching belts, the physios were smart in starched white but medical students, unless in operating gowns, shambled around the ward in ordinary clothes. It was probably a subtle way of making us aware that we were of less value than the dust as far as ward sisters were concerned.

It was also apt to cause confusion among patients as to who we actually were, as we never thought to introduce ourselves as we waded in to ask the most intimate questions and perform the most unseemly examinations. The patients, who had first thought that we were wandering out-of-hours visitors, became more and more confused. Consideration of patients, on reflection, was not the strong point of teaching hospitals in those days. Patients were necessary for the teachers and the taught but they had to know their place, which was unprotesting beneath the nice clean bedclothes; and woe betide the patient who turned his sheets grey from reading a freshly printed newspaper before a consultant's round; Sister would probably have asked for him to be discharged on the spot, or even worse – ordered an enema.

The only way for we mufti-clad students to establish our bona fides was to decorate ourselves with a stethoscope (not even lapel labels had been invented then). Thankfully, stethoscopes could be flourished. Alternatively, they could be dangled from pockets or, for the woman student, drooped as nonchalantly from the handbag as a Sloane Ranger allows her Liberty scarf to flow today. Thus we proved to the sceptical that we were indeed doctors in embryo. Unfortunately, it was brought to our attention that we were actually meant to put the stethoscopes to some other use than the purely decorative: we were to listen intelligently through them. The more mechanically minded among us had already discovered that they were excellent for tracing faults in car engines and for studying misbehaving household plumbing but, when applied to the chest, it became apparent that the wretched things did not supply automatic answers.

Breathing sounds were not too difficult to deal with but the trouble started with hearts. You had to listen, think, reason and then, horror of horrors, declare before a critical audience what you thought you had heard. It could expose you to horrible ridicule when it became apparent that the noises which travelled along your stethoscope tubing seemed to be quite different and always inferior to those which travelled along everyone else's.

Lub-dub, lub-dub we were told was the key to it all. Get that in your heads and you have the heart sounds. *Lub-dub, lub-dub,* who can go wrong? The answer could be anyone trying to hear anything at all through the hairy chest of a London docker, well padded with three inches of subcutaneous beer. The registrar will, however, make a point of the fact that he has heard perfectly, though heaven knows how. The consultant naturally will not admit that he cannot hear anything so moves hastily on to ridicule. After all, he has a sitting target, the butt of all jokes, the poor ward clerk. No consultant can lose face before juniors: playful witticisms concerning cabbages growing in students' ears fall from his exalted lips, always good for sycophantic laughter.

The basic mastery of *lub-dub* is not enough. The next step is murmurs. *Lub-shush-dub-rumble*. With a little practise even these extra noises could usually be fitted in but opening clicks and third split heart sounds were just plain unfair. Did they really exist or were they figments of the imagination of this same registrar who, aware that his chief was high-tone deaf, took great delight in expounding on them? At this stage the chief would be reduced to nodding in agreement with whatever his registrar said. He would be exactly imitated by the students, sinkingly aware of coffee-time coming and going and their feet hurting.

At St Elsewhere's, no-one sat during rounds, a sign of unimaginable weakness. Only once did a brave soul have the temerity to suggest that we should 'take a seat'. Perhaps he was already sure that he wanted to spend his life after qualification treating the natives in outer Bogdolia. 'Can we sit down, please Sir?' The words came wearily during a brief pause for breath taken by the wordiest and most boring registrar in the hospital. It was about as astounding as Oliver Twist asking for more.

The registrar had expounded for at least an hour and a quarter on the more obscure points of the heart sounds of poor Mr Willoughby, who was obviously now feeling considerably ` nearer to death than the recovery he had thought he was effecting before he was lighted on as an 'ideal teaching case'. From that moment he was paralysed on his pillow in rigid fear by the torrent of words which flowed over him. 'Risk of fatal arrhythmia . . . plah . . . plah . . . plah . . . oedema likely . . . cerebal confusion . . . scrape out the artery . . . ', and so on and on. Still Mr Willoughby stayed the course. At least he did not faint as did the patient whose keen attendant surgical registrar stood over him and said to the assembled students, 'Right boys, is he ready for the chop-chop?'

At the foot of Mr Willoughby's bed we students stood shifting uncomfortably from foot to foot. Actually it was less in discomfort and more in agony for some of us, as this was the stiletto heel era, but the men must have been pretty desperate, too, as it was a man who spoke. Evidently we women were made of sterner stuff.

The registrar paused momentarily in his flow of words. 'Certainly', he said benignly, 'Do sit!' Swiftly he seized the only available chair, sat on it firmly and continued to talk nonstop for another half hour. No-one asked again.

Heart surgery made its debut at this time and the consultant surgeons in this department became great gods. Wards were hushed and reverent when they entered with their entourage. A man who could operate on the heart of man! What power! Some had been interviewed on radio and television! We basked in a little reflected glory; after all, we trod the same wards: what kudos we gained among non-medical friends by talking about the feats of heart surgery almost as though we had performed the deeds ourselves. The fact that the nearest we got to a heart operation was the packed theatre gallery where the view was mostly of a sea of intent green surgically capped heads and complicated blood-slopping machines was not mentioned. We knew when we had an audience gripped.

Anaesthetists, too, came up into the league of folk heros at this time. Those who worked with the heart team strode with their masters, the technological wizards of the age. They had their moments of panic, however. Envisage an operation in its final stages. The chief anaesthetist has slipped away for a few minutes . . . important business . . . cup of tea . . . chat with Sister . . . who knows? Minions have been doing most of the work, in any case. The patient is moved on to the trolley to begin her journey back to the ward. Suddenly an urgent cry for oxygen goes up. The anaesthetist, refreshed, has wandered back into theatre and given the patient a cursory check. Her nails are purple! Terminal cyanosis! What could these juniors be thinking of to allow a patient out of theatre in this state? Whose heads will roll?

Closer inspection reveals nail varnish of a fashionable blue-black shade. The anaesthetist, not far from a heart attack himself, visions of his career in ruins having obviously passed through his head at tremendous speed, issues forth an edict. No nail varnish of any sort to be worn by patients in theatre. One more lowly job for the student clerking the patient. 'Your nail varnish must come off, Mrs Bloggs, otherwise the anaesthetist will not know if you are alive or dead': very reassuring information for the patient.

At last we were due to qualify and of course should have known all about hearts by then. Still, patients eager to help did not come amiss in Finals . . . I was doubly blessed. My first rose with a little bow as I came into his cubicle. He was more immaculate than the most immaculate consultant ever to be seen. His hair was trimmed and tidy to perfection. His hands were exquisite in their cleanliness and his dressing robe was tied with just that slight touch of nonchalance which imparts impeccable style. Reaching into his pocket he took out a neatly folded piece of paper. Written on it in immaculate copperplate writing was:

'Name – Willoughby Clarke.

Profession – gentleman's gentleman.

Purpose of visit – to demonstrate aortic valve leakage'.

He smiled gently. 'I don't like to see young ladies and gentlemen having difficulty and becoming confused', he said. 'If you will kindly listen here', pointing to the upper part of his chest, 'you may find it relevant to the present circumstances.'

Next I progressed to a mother and her small daughter. They were beaming happily. 'Ruth looks fine', I said to her mother, 'What is the trouble?' 'Oh', her mother said, 'It's just something that hasn't closed up in heart yet. The doctors say that it will be quite all right but it makes an interesting noise like machinery. Just listen there and you'll hear it.'

Safely qualified, it becomes evident that in the world of general practice the stethoscope remains a symbol, but here also it becomes the key to many doors, particularly those of old ladies. Anyone with a stethoscope must be all right for he cares for the heart and it's the heart that keeps you going, so the logic seems to run. Martha may have been living behind her chained front door in freezing squalor with her twelve cats for many weeks, defying the efforts of home helps and social workers who wish to enter. They may all fail to gain admission but as the bearer of a stethoscope, of no use for feeding or cleaning, warming or washing you will be beckoned in with a crafty smile. You are very welcome. Martha knows what is good for her.

In the surgery it can also rarely be used to full advantage without the maximum of fuss. The patients are free-spirited and are no longer firmly organised by Sister for 'the Round'. At last one appreciates the past efforts of nursing staff, which ensured that nightgowns and pyjama jackets were ready to be raised on command. Away from hospital, the twin gods of modesty and heat preservation reign supreme and the doctor is in luck who is at first request offered more than two square inches of upper chest wall on which to apply his bell or diaphragm. Dresses will, of course, open only at the back by complicted means, if then, and are too tight to raise above the waist. Palissades of elastic and lace, vests, lumbar corsets, pullovers, mysterious all-in-one garments bar the way. The ultimate challenge, though, is surprisingly not in the old but in the very young.

Master Matthew Puke is sure to be dressed in a tight-necked jumper which needs levering over his howling head and an impenetrable one-piece garment poppered deeply and un-reachably at the crutch. He has been brought by his father who has not a clue about how the whole thing works and who plonks him soggily on your knee when you say that you must listen to his heart.

Harold smugly presented a flash of hair chest, undoing his middle two shirt buttons and opening up a neat little diamond shape. 'Ho, ho, doctor,' he said, 'I'm not one of those who thinks their heart is round the side so just the middle here will do you, won't it?'

It all seems a silent conspiracy among the brotherhood of patients. Even when positively inviting you to listen with a re-mark such as, 'Perhaps you could just see if the old ticker is still turning over, doctor?' only the regulation miniscule amount of chest will be bared except, of course, when you have decided that it is really not necessary to make too much of an examina-tion and that your laying-on of stethoscope will be more for psychotherapeutic reasons than otherwise. In these cir-cumstances, however, do attend a little to what is happening. A colleague was somewhat discomfited to be asked, as he held his stethoscope bell to the chest wall of a persistent, neurotic patient nodding wisely but reflexly over a patient's heart, 'Don't you usually put the other bits in your ears, doctor?'

It is a great truth that, by the law of opposites, on the occa-sions when one does not really want to listen extensively the whole chest will be instantaneously bared. Often its owner will have come to the surgery especially bra-less to facilitate this event, or the male will throw off layers of black leather and teeshirt in no time at all to reveal his chest splendidly decor-ated with tattoos and gold medallions. Usually these patients will smell and one would rather not have come too close. But the 'heart concealer' is most definitely the more frequent bird of call. I try presenting an analogy with a motor car. 'How can a mechanic know what is going on in the engine if you don't open the bonnet right up?' I give what I hope is an encouraging little smile. This makes the patient give a nervous giggle (must laugh at doctor's little joke) but no more chest is bared.

A strange exception to my rule of 'however much you want to listen to the chest, the more obstacles will be put in your way' is Dora, an otherwise modest maiden lady with a heartbeat of outstanding irregularity. This has proved most difficult to put in order and has led to her making frequent visits to the surgery over many years for assessment of the results of the latest attempts to control it. Dora must have been very well schooled by a predecessor of mine in the practice as to what examination would be necessary on her visits and also as to how busy doctors are. She is so considerate of not wasting a moment of our precious time that on every occasion she leaps to her feet when called from the waiting room and stunningly comes in with one arm out of her blouse and cardigan and her elderly bosom already partially bared. Bodice-ripping has nothing on this. The rest of the waiting room is agog. 'I don't want to take up your time. I know that you will want to listen, doctor!' she says with a righteous smile.

Dora survived but I am given to understand that another elderly lady fared less well under my care. She puffed into the surgery saying she had been a little more breathless than usual for a few days. I asked her to climb onto the couch and undress so that I could listen to her heart. Five minutes later it became clear that it would be impossible to do that on this day. She did not feel that she could remove her corset. I made what I thought was a reasonable suggestion since she did not look particularly ill. 'Could you come back and see me tomorrow without your corset on, Mrs Grundy, and I will examine you then?' She nodded with what I thought was acquiescence but she never came back. A few weeks later I heard from another patient that she had collapsed while shopping and died. 'Her husband said it was because you told her that she must never wear her corset again and so she never did and you can't expect someone to manage after all those years, can you?' said my informant reproachfully. My reputation had taken a downturn in the neighbourhood.

No doctor gets it right every time, neither with patients nor with themselves. Dr D, who had suffered from a myocardial infarct some years before and so thought he knew all about these things in both a professional and personal way, went on holiday to France. Gripped with severe central chest pain as he was driving home he confidently diagnosed 'another coronary' but was blowed if he was going to be ill in a 'damned Frog hospital'. Gritting his teeth he drove onto the car ferry; clutching his chest he survived the crossing; a short drive on the home side of the Channel, and he was in a good old English casualty department. The most senior emergency medical staff were hastily mobilised to deal with this suffering fellow doctor. His shirt was tenderly opened by the consultant he had come so far to find. Out fell a dead wasp. Just another example of how we get things wrong. We do, all the time; the only consolation is that on occasions it gives patients a chance to gloat, but if we are smug we will certainly get our come-uppance.

Mrs Field scored a notable victory for patients recently in the subtle contest that goes on between patients and their medical advisors and left me checking and rechecking any dismissive diagnosis I had been tempted to make of a cardiac problem since I saw her.

She looked remarkably cheerful when she came in to the surgery one Monday morning. She was last in from the waiting room but I was not destined to have my coffee for some time. I hopefully thought that she might be beaming because I had at last found some cure for her usual complaints of aching feet and weeping ulcers, but it was not so. First, I heard about my failure and how my latest efforts had been even less effective than usual. Nothing unusual. However, this was not all I was to hear that morning. I evidently needed to be given a fine example of the patient as diagnostician. It was all to do with her neighbour's doctor. Mrs Field had seen her neighbour, Mr Birtenshaw, looking poorly when she met him hobbling from his front door for his milk as she emerged from her own front door across the landing to do the same. 'I took one look at him and told him he needed his doctor', she said with relish. 'I knew that look he had about him. It was just like my poor Bert. Of course you never met my poor Bert, doctor. He was gone before your time. Married him after three days I did when my mother had my wedding all arranged for next week with Pete. Bit annoyed my mum was with the reception all being wasted like because I just went off and married Bert on the quiet, like, but we were ever so happy and my mum took to Bert in the end and so we didn't do too badly. Twenty-five years I was married to him. Anyway, doctor, one morning Bert looked really queer but he told me to get along and go to the hairdresser's because I was booked all up to have a perm because it was special half price that week and we had a wedding on Saturday. My cousins you know, doctor, that went to Australia and then she came back with the children again because she never got properly settled and her Ken met this Doreen. You remember the Kellys who lived at number 25, don't you, doctor. Well, their stepson's second wife had this daughter', I must have looked a little confused at this point, 'and well I won't hold you up any more doctor but the next thing when I came back from having my hair done there were just a pair of feet sticking out of the kitchen and that was the end of Bert. His heart, you know!' The epic continued.

'Anyway I saw my neighbour again at lunchtime because he put the cat out and I said to him you look rough and he said he was OK and I said he didn't look right to me and if he wasn't going to call the doctor I would, and he said he wasn't but I could if I liked so I did. I rang the receptionist and told her to get that doctor down fast and she argued a bit but I heard him come and when he was going, I just happened to have my front door open, to let the air in you know, doctor, and I just happened to hear him say "When you want the doctor, you call him yourself next time and don't let any interfering old busybody call him for you. You're fine, old chap." '

Mrs Field did not appear at all offended at the slight cast on her. She knew her best lines were to come. Her nostrils merely twitched with contempt for the doctor who did not know a heart patient when he saw one. 'Anyway next day, that was Sunday you know, I thought I would just pop in to see how Mr Birtenshaw was and there was no reply when I knocked at the door and I knew that he couldn't have gone out or I would have heard him. So I called my neighbour and she knocked too but it was all quiet inside so we rang his nephew and he came up from the country with his key but the door was bolted so he got the police and the fire brigade to get in and there was Mr Birtenshaw dead in bed. It was his heart you know. I knew the look!'

I wished that I was such a confident and accurate diagnostician, but hearts are always a puzzle.

ANN WHITEHEAD

London

Houseman Hearts, or Tickers to Remember

Although my first pre-registration post was entitled General Surgery, at the Royal Infirmary, Glasgow, there was more to it than that. Three months on the busy professorial general unit was followed by six weeks in genito-urinary work and then to six energy- and emotion-sapping weeks in a small but progressive cardiac surgery unit, where Professor William Arthur Mackey and Mr Bill Bain were well to the fore in specialist techniques. This was in 1963 and although a central intensive care unit for the hospital had recently opened the cardiac unit did its own special care in the unit which was across the courtyard (or through the tunnel) from the main hospital. The house surgeon slept there all the time and there was a second room which a duty SHO or registrar could use on immediate post-operative nights.

One night, a lady who had been in theatre for a mitral valvotomy earlier in the day began to twitch and had unusual features on her ECG. Our own biochemist was mustered and she could not detect any deficiencies in the samples. Senior help was called for; a variety of anti-arrhythmic agents were tried; eventually after a bolus of phenytoin the twitching stopped and the ECG reverted to what we would have expected from such a patient. We felt well pleased with our efforts and turned in to get some sleep. It was mid-morning the following day when the patient's full case notes arrived from her referring hospital, and before adding them to the folder of technical cardiology notes I read them. Lo and behold, I discovered that her mitral valve problem had been detected when she had been admitted to a district hospital after having had a fit in the street. She had in fact been suffering from epilepsy for many years but had never been good at following her recommended therapy, had no card or explanatory note with her, and all through the investigation stage had never mentioned it. Her general practitioner had been informed by letter at each stage but had never responded with any comment . . . perhaps in that practice, at that time, all letters were simply filed by the clerical staff. Despite the information gap the patient did well and was soon discharged to lead a new and friskier life.

I moved to Stobhill hospital for my six months as a House physician with Dr J.B. Rennie. This hospital was a series of spread-out two-story units and a resuscitation procedure was just being established. A designated team had not yet been formed nor had 'bleeps' of any sort yet been provided. When a cardiac arrest occurred, the switchboard put out a coded message over the general loudspeaker system and it was expected that almost any free junior doctors would respond and rush to the labelled ward. One evening, such a call came and off we went. We tore into the ward and found a tiny little Glasgow man lying on his bed shouting for help. Leaning over him and semi-wrapped around him while she pummelled his chest was a full bosomed, long-haired final year student who was doing a short locum. We disentangled the apparently fit patient from her tresses and found that the main connection of the cable to the ECG machine had slipped out. Patient and assailant soon recovered. This was one of a series of episodes that led to a mammoth meeting of most of the hospital staff and resulted in the formation of a resuscitation team and a back-up policy.

Individual medical wards did not have their own ECG machine and during the daytime a team of gorgeous lassies pushed the official machine around the hospital and performed all the routine ECGs. On St Valentine's Day they arrived on the ward on what seemed a routine visit, but all three were there and one was carrying a large brown hospital envelope. This was handed to me and inside was the most original Valentine I have ever seen. By using various cuts and traces and pasting these onto card, they had selected ones to say 'you make our hearts go . . . ' Perhaps the rhythm that they finished with is better left unsaid, but I can assure you that the link with that fine team, blossomed over the rest of my time at Stobhill.

A colleague on another ward was an attractive and neat girl from Kenya who proudly wore her national dress when at work in the wards. Over it she wore a white coat, but as usual buttons were often missing. There was not yet a coronary care unit and all patients were cared for in the ordinary wards. At that time, it was felt that all post-infarct patients should have blood pressure readings that showed they were doing well; this was not always easy to achieve and all sorts of nasty chemicals were available for injecting to try to get the readings up. Dr Rogan, for whom this lady worked, was an astute and observant doctor and after a while he realised that whenever she measured a man's blood pressure the results seemed higher than he could achieve. He spent a long time watching her and eventually he spotted that her best results were on the days that she wore a buttonless white coat and that it was the eye-level view of her silky brown skin which had the excellent effect on the little Glasgow men with heart attacks. Understandably, once he started boasting to his colleagues about his new form of 'pressor therapy', the good lady was in great demand from all quarters and at all hours.

I had worked at the Evelina Children's Hospital of Guy's Hospital in 1964 as paediatric house officer and though I had been very much aware of Lord Brock at Guy's and had seen him, I did not actually meet him then. I returned to Guy's in 1966 to one of the SHO posts in the Nuffield, or private wing. Lord Brock was one of the consultants who used the wing and he performed some cardiac surgery in the small theatre there. I heard one day that he was to do a mitral valvotomy so I asked if I could observe. He welcomed me warmly, and like any good teacher determined my knowledge of the procedure before explaining what he had done so far, giving me a summary of the patient's history. He became excited when I said that not only had I seen the Brock mitral valve dilator used, but had assisted Professor William Arthur Mackey at operations in Glasgow when he had been using it. As the operation progressed he carefully explained each stage and at the end was most profuse in thanking me for my interest. Over the following six months, there were several occasions when he was short of one of his regular assistants and I would be asked if I could go to the theatre to help.

On about the 29th of each month, his secretary would telephone and ask me to confirm that I had assisted him on particular dates. On the following day a welcome cheque would arrive. I doubly welcomed the cheque, the kind thoughts and the courtesy that accompanied it as I knew that north of the river there were at that time senior registrars in cardiac surgery and anaesthetics who did an immense amount more for the patients of other cardiac surgeons who did not seem to receive even a token. I was due to move to another hospital on the following 1 January, but in mid-December received an invitation for myself and a partner to the famous Lord Brock Hogmanay party in Wimbledon. This was a marvellous evening given for all his staff but I had thought that I was too much on the fringe, and itinerant, to be considered 'staff'. Midnight struck and the staff let loose all the suppressed feelings of the year with much shouting and bursting of balloons. Lord Brock sidled over to my partner and me, apologised for the way they had all exploded and said that he hoped that the noise would not upset the thoughts and feelings that he was aware Scottish people had at the 'Turn of the Year'.

One evening in Stobhill Hospital in Glasgow we had a burly man who complained of chest pain, and despite apparent changes on his ECG my colleagues and I were not convinced that he had just had a heart attack, as he was claiming. In 1964, we had no rapid cardio-enzyme test available so it seemed that we would need to take him into one of our few empty beds. However, we surreptiously searched his jacket pockets and there we found an appointment card for the Southern General Hospital, which was across the other side of town. We rang them to see if they would look out his old notes, and to our surprise we found that he had been in their department with a similar story that evening. By checking times in detail, we found that because of intermittent buses on two 'dog-leg' routes the only way he could have got to us so soon was by taxi. Intrigued as we were with his actions and his story, we gently eased him back towards the City of Glasgow. The sequel to this was that some four years later, when working in Lewisham Hospital, London, I was called to give an opinion on a man from Glasgow with an abnormal ECG. To my surprise, it was the same fellow and after I had explained where and how we had met before, he once again departed quietly into the night. His name and description were added to the fascinating 'black book' that was kept there and I often wonder what happened to the book and whether, one day, someone will bother to publish it.

Some years later I had responsibility for the resuscitation team at the Middlesex Hospital in the centre of London. We had become despondent about our success rate of reviving 'arrested hearts' brought in by ambulance. We had a good team and had just been permitted the purchase of a fine new machine, which was one of the first that enabled the reading of an ECG by simply holding the paddles on the chest, so that a shock could be immediately given if required.

One day, a taxi driver was brought in and the ambulance crew explained that they had been cruising along a nearby street when they were waved down. The taxi driver had felt unwell, pulled into the side of the street and collapsed over his wheel. Luckily, a man trained in first aid had been on the pavement and seen it happen. He pulled the driver from his cab and gave cardiac massage, which was continued in the ambulance. We had been called and were waiting at the door of the casualty department. Our fine new machine worked and the patient was soon in a ward upstairs. Physically, he made tremendous progress but to our great disappointment his memory and reasoning abilities lagged behind. On one of my visits to his ward I was thrilled to see that he was reading a newspaper but alas, when I got closer, I found that it was upside down. Transfer to a rehabilitation unit was arranged, but as they did not want him to be transferred until after the imminent public holiday it was arranged that he would go home for the weekend. He was then to return to us on the following Tuesday morning as his transfer had to be from ward to ward. When he returned I happened to be standing in the front hall as he came through the door. I saw his wife point him towards me and over he came, saying my name and effusing his thanks for all that we had done for him. A few minutes' conversation established that he was fully back in touch with life, so we just turned him around, sent him back home with his wife and found another patient to use his place in the rehabilitation unit.

In my sixteen years in Isolated Island Practice, despite the fact that for the last few years I have had both a partner and a trainee, it has nevertheless transpired that more often than not I have been on duty over Christmas Eve. However, this was the first year that I had not been in the house for the so-exciting moment when the family attacked their Christmas stockings. This year was to have been rather important, as it appeared that it would be the last year when our youngest son was to be a 'believer'. We were suspicious of his belief as, when he wrote his letter to Santa in November and had put it up the chimney, he had refused to let either of us read it. We had seen him studying several mail-order catalogues but we were stuck when it came to trying to spot what he was keen on, as he had not marked any of the pages. However, our luck was in. We live in a windy spot and the 82-year-old chimney has no modern narrow lining and is quite wide, with many irregular and rough patches. An outer door was opened, and as the peat fire had died a little the down-draught brought the letter back onto the hearth, still readable. We were able to shop accordingly. It now became vital that we were there to observe his response.

Alas, it was not to be. The phone rang at 0600 hrs and was a elderly lady who lived 15 miles away, saying her husband had a terrible pain in his chest and looked very unwell. Clinical and electromechanical assessment confirmed my own and the lady's fear. The nurse had arrived so we gradually made him comfortable and arranged a visiting schedule for the rest of the day. Leaving the lady and her husband in the care of a nephew whom we had summoned, the nurse and I set off for our homes.

Initially I was simply heading home, but on the way and before I reached the main junction, I realised that it was now 0800
hrs and I had missed youngest son and his thrill. However, I
had been out during the previous evening to visit the younger
of two small boys who had been unwell. I had promised the
family that I would visit again at about 0900 hrs and now
realised that they would be up, as well, so I turned off in their
direction. On arrival at their house I found that the little fellow
was on the mend, so I was able to sit and savour the joy and delight with which the two little fellows explored and opened
their parcels. Home, then, to mounds of paper and boxes with,
fortunately, lots of excitement left in our own trio.

I suppose that, in some big mainland practices, these visits
would have been carried out by a deputising service and the
personal social disruption would not have occurred. However,
this day was rewarding and more than compensated for the
upsets.

JOHN MACLEOD

Isle of North Uist

The Marsh Quality of Life Profile

It was Galen who said that 'The chief merit of language is
clearness, and we know that nothing detracts so much from
this as do unfamiliar terms'. Now, I am not unfamiliar with the
terms 'Quality of Life' or 'Quality of Life profile', but I am not
sure that I know what they actually mean. They are definitely,
however, the 'buzz-words' of the moment, just as 'buzz-
words' are 'buzz-words' *ad infinitum*.

But Quality of Life – what does it really mean? Having plenty
of money? food? a good home? Or is it having a hangover or
indigestion or headache? Is it only associated with old age, or
chronic disease, or cancer? Should every doctor experience it
before he or she can talk about it? I certainly know more about

the need to examine a broken finger or limb gently after suffering that fate myself. Similarly, I am now much more aware of the wretched feeling and fear associated with lobar pneumonia. I was especially struck with my bronchial breathing sounding as if I had organ pipes inserted into my chest, and the consequent delight of knowing that the antibiotic had reached the cause of the problem (to places other antibiotics cannot reach) when I experienced an unmistakable penicillinic acid taste in my sputum.

So how can one get to know more about Quality of Life? Simple – have a myocardial infarction. In fact, have a massive infarction, be admitted to a coronary care unit and then have asystole while your physician and cardiologist are standing at the bottom of the bed deciding what to do. That is also a good way to get them to experience a few ectopics themselves, not to mention other potential disasters. Once you have been resuscitated and transferred to the regional cardiothoracic unit, had a pacing wire inserted and been admitted to the intensive care unit, I suggest you quietly develop septicaemia. A methicillin-resistant staphylococcus would be interesting. This often leads to bacterial endocarditis, destruction of the heart valves, heart failure and, if you are lucky, the insertion of an aortic balloon pump. What next? Well, how about a heart transplant? After all, you are in Harefield Hospital and it would be silly to miss the opportunity. After that it is easy – over 12 kg loss in weight, learning to walk again, lifelong anti-rejection therapy, regular screening for signs of rejection and slowly back to work six months later. For this you get a Quality of Life questionnaire to fill in – if you make it.

The one I had is called the Nottingham Health Profile, and was probably instituted when Robin Hood was trying to make up his mind whether he would rather have his way with Maid Marion in Sherwood Forest or on a nice comfortable bed in Nottingham General Hospital. There are six question topics – physical mobility, pain, energy, social isolation, emotional reactions and sleep. Most questions were quite easy to answer. I was becoming more mobile, the pain was decreasing, energy increasing, I was not isolated but I did have an emotional reaction – I was not too happy, to put it mildly, at having had to

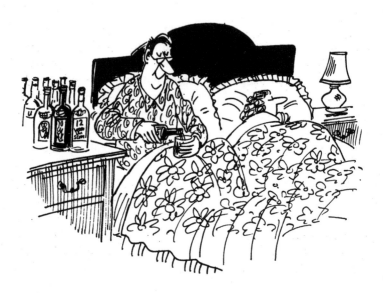

I am prepared to carry on experimenting until I am sure the profile is reproducible and repeatable.

have a heart transplant. Sleep was my real problem, however. In the profile, there are five questions on sleep – basically they are about early wakening, difficulty in getting off to sleep, sleeping badly, use of sleeping tablets and staying awake most of the night. My problem was in trying to make my answers fit the questions. I had no difficulty in dropping off to sleep, but woke up several times during the night, usually, not always, managing to sleep again each time. Notice the difficulty I was in? I have already described a different problem to any of the questions in the profile. My problem was in sleeping the second, third or fourth time around and it was harder each time I awoke. I know, in fact, why I have this problem, but the Nottingham Health Profile is not sophisticated enough to bring out this reason.

Before my operation I slept on my right side. Now, because of discomfort following sternal division and subsequent minor, but noticeable to me, instability of the union, I sleep on my back. So I snore – and my wife wakes me because she cannot sleep. I have partially cured the problem by giving her some ear plugs, but there is yet another problem. I take cyclosporin to prevent rejection. It is nephrotoxic. Despite being on a relatively low dose, I have developed mild renal failure with a regular nocturia, responsive to several inter-related factors. The higher the dose of cyclosporin, the more often I have to get up at night and vice versa. As luck would have it, I have been able to overcome this side effect with the judicious use of another drug – alcohol. Suitable draughts of this drug appear to narcotise the bladder distension receptors, at least until a reasonable time in the morning. Nevertheless, if I make an error in the dose more difficulties arise. Too low a dose allows the diuretic effects of the alcohol to overcome the sedative effects. Conversely, too high a dose increases the snoring decibel level so penetrating my wife's earplugs and invoking a painful and awakening dig in the ribs. I did for a short time examine the effects of alcohol on my wife's hearing. However, when she spontaneously remarked that she could not tell the difference between the cheapest scotch and the best, I abandoned that study and bought her another pair of earplugs.

In the meantime, I am conducting the Marsh Quality of Life Profile. I too have five groups – Islay, Highland, Speyside, Island (Jura, Mull, Orkney, Skye) and others. As you may by now have realised, they are all regions of malt whisky manufacture. My profile is based on four questions – taste, amount needed to prevent recurrent awakening, effect upon wife's sleeping pattern and a cost/benefit analysis, i.e., can I afford the treatment?

I am prepared to carry on experimenting until I am sure the profile is reproducible and repeatable. It could take many years – I hope. After all, research is never-ending and we never know when we have all the answers. My local wine merchant stocks over 50 malts and there are at least another 50 out there waiting to be discovered. I think that I am slowly but surely coming to understand what Quality of Life means. One thing is certain – it is definitely different now to what it was before my 'transplant', both in fact and in attitude. I am ever more certain that no Quality of Life profile will give a true and absolute measure of how a patient feels, but what is absolute in this world anyway? So I reckon my Quality of Life profile is as good as any of the others and here's health to Harefield

Hospital, Magdi Yacoub and the Marsh Quality of Life research programme.

B.T. MARSH

Chalfont St Peter

Cardiac *Faux Pas*

On my first day in America, horribly jet-lagged in the torrid southern heat, I went to the pool. It was full of delectable ladies whose bikinis seemed to be made of string and three postage stamps. Nothing was left to my imagination. This was trying for a middle-aged Englishman doing his poor best breast stroke.

On day two I was in the clinic, frightened witless by all things strange, especially the language and culture. I soon discovered that female patients prepared for the doctor by removing their clothes and donning an examination gown. These are made of paper and, like operating gowns, invest everything except face, hands and feet. The ladies, now ready for anything that the doctor might do, were more covered up than when they walked in from the street, and revealed infinitely less than when at the pool.

The first morning was difficult. I soon tired of asking how to manage problems, from switching on lights (the wrong way), flushing loos and trying to understand what that drawl which passes for speech in the Southern States really meant. Suddenly there was an emergency. An elderly black woman had acute chest pain and temporarily the Real Doctor was missing. In such a crisis even the strange Limey, alleged to be a physician, might do. An urgent young nurse bustled me to the paper-cocooned lady. Fearing to ask yet again what to do, I seized the patient's gown at the collar and tore, revealing all to the navel. A sharp intake of breath made me glance up. The nurse's eyes informed me of impossible solecism. If she had been drawn in a comic-strip cartoon there would have been a

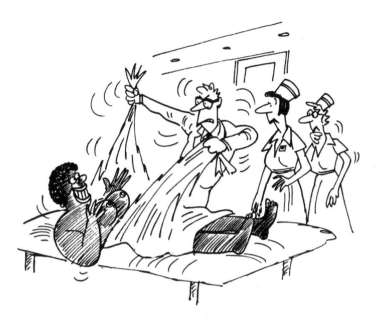

He don't look much but he's all man!

speech balloon protruding from her head saying 'My Gard, we got a rapist . . .'.

The situation was saved by the patient. Turning to the nurse she observed: 'He don't look much, but he's all man.'

ROBIN HULL

Birmingham

Sing a Song

Sing a song of sixpence,
   Our bread is made of rye,
Four and twenty carrots
   Baked in a pie,
No butter in the pastry,
   No salt to give it taste –
It hasn't got much flavour
   But does wonders for your waist.

The king was in his multi-gym, his muscles getting sorer,
The queen was in the kitchen, eating bread* and Flora,
The maid was in the garden, jogging round and round
Until she sprained her ankle and fell to the ground.

The neighbours heard her shouting, a doctor came and then
He fixed her leg with Tubigrip and off she went again.

*(wholemeal, of course)

MARIE CAMPKIN
London

5
The Medical History of a Great Musician

Illness, especially fatal illness, in famous people is an interesting branch of medical history. It is often a study in detection based on slender strands of contemporary evidence, and may be little more than barely informed guesswork. More reliable information is often available concerning men of distinction and genius of recent times. Particular attention has been paid to the health of world political leaders and its possible effect on national and international affairs. One submission to this series was an account of the illness which caused the death of Gustav Mahler. He died from infective endocarditis before effective treatment was available.

Directly from his Inmost Heart

Into the opening bars of his Ninth Symphony Gustav Mahler pulsed the irregular rhythm of his own failing heart. He died in Vienna on 18 May, 1911, after a final illness as dramatic as any opera.

Mahler met Alma Schindler on 7 November, 1901. He proposed within three weeks of their first meeting; they were engaged before Christmas, married before Easter, parents before a year had passed.

During their courtship Mahler once tore open his shirt, bared his chest and pressed Alma's hand upon his heart. But the gesture was romantic, not diagnostic: in 1901 Mahler was in robust good health, an enthusiast for bicycling, rowing, under-water swimming and mountaineering.

So powerful was his presence that Gustav Klimt painted his likeness as 'the Well-armed Strong One' in his enormous allegorical Beethoven frieze for the 1902 Sezession Exhibition. An heroic knight in gilded armour strides purposefully to-

wards a large group of 'Hostile Forces' – assorted ladies repre-
senting Lust, Lewdness and other picturesque vices – his
stylished profile an unmistakable portrait of Mahler. At forty-
one he was the virtual dictator of the Vienna Opera, sought as
conductor throughout Europe and feted as a composer of
increasing influence. Alma Schindler was twenty-two, beautiful, captivating, courted by the artistic leaders of the Austro-
Hungarian capital. She too had been painted by Klimt, but his
feeling for her was more compelling and less cerebral than his
admiration for Mahler. He had abandoned his canvasses to follow her to Italy, only to be sent packing by her mother, who
exercised her maternal solicitude by reading her daughter's
diaries.

Soon after their marriage Mahler wrote to Alma, 'I should
like now to have success, recognition, and all those other really
quite meaningless things people talk of. I want to do you
honour.' She appreciated his concern. She told him later, 'All
I love in a man is his achievement. The greater his achievement
the more I have to love him.' There were achievements in
plenty. Much of the year was spent in a hectic round of opera
productions, rehearsals and performances at the Imperial
Court Opera House. Its orchestra, trooping up from the Opera
House pit to the concert platform, reassembled as the Vienna
Philharmonic and played again under Mahler's baton. He
travelled to all points of the compass to conduct concerts in
Europe's most appreciative and most demanding venues:
Helsinki, Rome, Cologne, Strasbourg, Weimar, Basel, Amster-
dam. The journeys alone would have exhausted weaker
constitutions.

He did, however, have a weakness: he suffered from tonsillitis throughout his life. Even on his honeymoon – a conducting tour to St Petersburg – he caught a chill on the train. He
arrived feverish, too hoarse to raise his voice above a croak. In
childhood he developed St Vitus's Dance, which left him with
involuntary movements of his right leg, and an irregular gait.
Colleagues mistook the tapping of his foot as an impatient
fidget, a perfectionist fret of temper, or a nervous tic. It had
more serious implications: it was a marker of the rheumatic
damage which had also scarred the valves of his heart.

Before his marriage Mahler had built himself a lakeside re-treat at Maiernigg in Carinthia, a spot hand-picked for him by a nesting soprano. Each summer he took leave of Vienna and its incessant interpretations of the creations of others and turned instead to a season of personal creativity. Entirely absorbed in his composition every morning, he renewed his inspiration as he trekked in the high mountains through the rest of the long light days. This tradition continued after his marriage, a 'splendid isolation' eagerly shared by Alma and their two little daughters, who tiptoed and whispered in the mornings, then raced laughing through the countryside whenever Mahler emerged from his self-imposed seclusion.

He completed his Fifth Symphony during their first summer together, and his Sixth Symphony two years later. He was newly married to a young wife who returned his love, yet he was impelled to write this 'Tragic' Symphony, which ends, as he explained to her, with 'three hammer blows of fate, which fell the hero as a tree is felled'. When he came to conduct the première in Essen in 1906, the bass drum was not loud enough for him: he had a huge wooden chest specially constructed, to intensify the boom of the fateful blows. The dress rehearsal moved him to uncontrollable sobs of dread. Later he found himself unable to listen to the third blow – the Death Blow – and removed it from the score. Alma recounted how she wept with him on the day he first played the completed work to her, understanding that it 'came directly from his inmost heart'.

But she was less understanding with his next opus. Mahler turned again to his settings of the poems written in mourning by Friedrich Ruckert – the magnificent and heartrending 'Kindertotenlieder' (Songs on the Death of Children). It was too much for Alma, who was still breast-feeding the baby Anna. 'For Heaven's sake,' she begged, 'don't tempt Fate'. Fate entered in the guise of a nanny.

In the Spring of 1904 Alma complained about 'a scatter-brained maid who literally expected me to wait upon her'. She was replaced. In 1906 they acquired a fashionably English, laudably long-serving children's nanny. They might have done better to appoint Typhoid Mary as the family cook, for this 'fussy English nurse' was subject to repeated septic sore throats.

After Easter 1907 Mahler conducted three concerts in Rome;
Alma went with him. On their return she found that the nurse
'had scalded three fingers of my younger child's hand . . . She
got feverish and sick – it was scarlet fever . . . ' Weeks went by
before the two-year-old Anna recovered her health and was released from quarantine. Her older sister Maria went to stay
with her Grandmother for safety. The family re-grouped for
their usual summer holiday at Maiernigg. Within three days
Maria fell ill with 'scarlet fever and diphtheria'. Soon her only
chance of survival was tracheotomy, a desperate attempt to
save her from choking to death. The English nurse helped to
set up the operating table, but the intervention was in vain.
Maria, only four years old, died on 12 July, 1907. Two days
later, catching sight of Maria's coffin as it was loaded into the
hearse, Alma swooned, and her mother collapsed with a heart
attack. The family doctor was summoned. As he finished his
assessment of Alma, Mahler said, 'Come along, Doctor, would
you like to examine me too?' Perhaps Dr Blumenthal resented
this Viennese variation of 'While you're here, Doctor . . .', for,
after applying his stethoscope, he blurted his opinion: 'You
have no cause to be proud of a heart like that.' Mahler's daughter lay unburied, his mother-in-law stricken and his wife in-
consolable. A non-committal comment might have sufficed
until after the funeral.

As soon as he could get away Mahler rushed to Vienna. A
cardiologist confirmed the diagnosis of rheumatic heart disease, ordered complete rest, forbade any exercise. Mahler was
horrified at this blanket restriction upon a central source of his
recuperative powers. His friend Bruno Walter recalled his des-
pairing fatalism: 'Accustomed to relying on long walks, even
on mountain climbing, for the inspiration of his music, he now
had to restrict all bodily movement as much as possible . . . his
world, his life lay under the sombre shadow . . .'

He continued his walks, but stopped every few yards to feel
his pulse, or to ask Alma to listen to his heart. He carried a
pedometer, counted his footsteps, timed his heartbeats. He assumed the worst: he was condemned to the life of a cripple; he
was in mortal danger. In an unsuccessful attempt to cancel a
series of concerts in St Petersburg, he wrote to Herr Schroder

– Royal Piano Maker and Concert Agency – 'This excessive exertion would, in view of a disease of the heart which set in this summer, make it very difficult for me to carry out my agreement. My doctor has absolutely forbidden me to undertake such exhausting journeys.' The concerts went ahead.

In any case, Mahler's idea of a complete rest was to sign a contract with the Metropolitan Opera House in New York; in three months he produced and conducted five operas. He returned to Austria for his customary summer of composition, avoiding the blighted Maiernigg and settling into an isolated farmhouse at Toblach in the Tyrol. He had completed his Eighth Symphony – the Symphony of a Thousand – in 1906, his 'last summer of peace, beauty and content'. He planned his next work as a 'Symphony of Songs'. Then, recalling the deaths of Beethoven and Bruckner after their Ninth Symphonies, he changed the title to 'The Song of the Earth'. When in 1911 he did complete his Ninth Symphony he told Alma, like a child comforted by crossed fingers, that it was really his Tenth, so the danger was past.

The danger came now from another direction. Alma went on a cure, and fell in love. Walter Gropius was young, handsome, talented, impetuous and ardent. He wrote to her at Toblach, protesting that he could not live without her and begging her to run away with him. He addressed the envelope, however, not to Alma, but to 'Herr Direktor Mahler'. Her husband's reaction was all Alma might have wished for. He loved her to distraction, to obsession. She woke in the night to find him standing mooning over her. He wrote her poems and passionate love letters. He enthused over songs she had composed years before, demanded extravagant praise of them from their friends.

The excitements continued. Gropius followed her to Toblach and skulked near the house. Alma spotted him and, far from sending him away, informed her desperate husband of the proximity of the rival who menaced his happiness. Mahler, ill with a further throat infection caught from the English nanny, summoned the young man into the drawing room, asked Alma to choose between them, and retired upstairs to await her decision. After deliberations lasting some hours, she resolved to resist Gropius's entreaties: she would stay with Mahler.

She saw Gropius off at the station. The train steamed away and so did Gropius, sending impassioned vows by telegram from every stop on his journey. Mahler, in a passion of fear lest she jump onto the train with the love-sick intruder, set off in another carriage to follow her. But Alma was satisfied. She was beloved not once, but twice. It was enough.

Mahler, however, was frantic. He submitted first to cauterisation of his tonsils, then to psychotherapy. He cabled Sigmund Freud, holidaying on the Baltic coast: Freud cabled an appointment: Mahler cabled a cancellation, then a second cancellation, then a third. Freud suggested a fourth date, his final offer. They met in Leiden in August, 1910, one month after Mahler's fiftieth birthday. Freud made his pronouncements: Mahler was obsessed with his mother; he called his wife Marie because that was his mother's name; he wished his wife to look careworn as she had done. However, whatever Mahler's faults, Freud predicted, Alma would stay with him, but with no credit to Mahler. Alma was merely fulfilling her subconcious need for her father, who had died when she was fourteen, the victim of a medical bungle – he had had the misfortune to develop acute appendicitis in the middle of a cholera epidemic.

Freud's theorising was attractive, but wrong. Alma was attracted to high achievers, not older men, and as for calling his wife by his mother's name, Maria happened to be Alma's middle name although Mahler never used it. He always called her by the Viennese diminutive, Almschli. It seems hardly tactful to have pointed out to Mahler that he was old enough to be his wife's father, just at the time when she had a devoted follower four years her junior. And if he knew of Gropius's love letter addressed to the unsuspecting husband he made no note of this Freudian slip. Whatever the quality of the advice, the transference was satisfactory. After the consultation he wrote to Alma: 'Eros is the ruler of men and gods . . . surely will I make a fresh conquest . . . of the heart which once was mine.' He returned to Vienna with renewed determination to satisfy Alma's needs, both mental and physical. For a man on the brink of cardiac failure, it must have been exhausting.

Alma, always an adept emotional extortionist, continued to extract proofs of his devotion. He dedicated his Eighth Symphony to her and wore her wedding ring during rehearsals, fighting through a further bout of tonsillitis. He conducted the triumphant première in Munich on 12 September, 1910. It was his last concert in Europe.

In the audience Thomas Mann was overcome by the occasion and the music. He was still lost for words when presented to Mahler after the concert, and wrote an effusive note to excuse himself for his gaucheness, enclosing a copy of his latest book. Mahler returned to America in November, 1910, contracted to conduct sixty-five concerts in New York, Buffalo, Springfield and Seattle. The incessant travel exhausted him: the interminable wrangling of the society ladies who ran the New York Philharmonic enraged him. The English nanny passed on another of her 'septic throats'. He became feverish while rehearsing for a concert at Carnegie Hall on 21 February, 1911. After the performance he took to his bed with a swinging temperature. His condition worsened, more prolonged and debilitating than any previous attack of tonsillitis.

His friend, Dr Joseph Fraenkel recognised the signs: Mahler had subacute bacterial endocarditis. Fraenkel was so grief-stricken at the diagnosis that his hair went white overnight. Unlike the brusque Dr Blumenthal he made reassuring comments, but he ordered the immediate preparation of blood cultures.

A doctor from the Montefiore Hospital prepared samples with the surgical finesse of an army barber, splashing blood around bedroom and bathroom of their ninth floor hotel suite. Mahler threatened to throw the next bungler down the stairs. The blood cultures yielded streptococci. The New York doctors injected Kollargol. There was no improvement. With no more to offer they encouraged Mahler to seek a cure among the bacteriologists of Europe. He and his family embarked at once. They arrived in Paris at Easter with their letters of referral. The celebrated doctors were away on holiday.

They called in Professor Andre Chantemesse of the Pasteur Institute, a man with the bedside manner of a B-movie boffin. He drew off further samples of Mahler's blood into culture bottles; when the results were ready he returned, elated, carrying a microscope. He summoned Alma and her mother to come and admire the slides he had prepared. Full of renewed hope for a cure, Alma looked through the eyepiece, then the horror dawned on her that the 'seaweed strands' in her field of view were signs of infection in her husband's bloodstream. Still Chantemesse enthused, 'Even I, myself, have never seen streptococci in such a marvellous state of development.' His sympathies clearly lay with the bacteria.

Alma telegraphed to Vienna for Professor Franz Chvostek, who took the next train for Paris. He saw at once that a cure was impossible, but that Mahler's morale might benefit from a move back to Vienna. Chvostek strengthened Mahler for the ordeal of the journey by implying that the illness was merely a breakdown due to overwork. He rallied briefly. He arrived at the Loew Sanatorium on 12 May to find his room filled with flowers. At first he was able to hold court in his room, but he rapidly weakened. His knee became swollen; he was treated by an application of radium; the swelling subsided. Daily, then hourly, bulletins announced the progress of his illness. Thomas Mann followed the newspaper reports as he holidayed in Italy during an outbreak of cholera. He was soon at work on 'Death in Venice', giving his protagonist, Aschenbach, the same appearance, the same age and even the same first name as his idol. Gustav Mahler.

As his strength waned, Mahler realised that he would compose no more. He gave Alma the unfinished manuscript of his Tenth Symphony. Across the final pages he had scrawled the desperate words:

> To live for you
> To die for you
> my Almschli.

He had spoken often in his last years of retiring to a house in the country, of ending the incessant travel, of saving his strength, of finding time for his composition, for living. Now there was no more time. He was suddenly tearful; 'My life has all been paper.' But he had at last achieved his childhood ambition: when he was only five years old someone had asked him what he wished to be when he grew up. His answer had been determined, and puzzling: 'A martyr.' He died six days later, while a thunderstorm raged outside. Again and again he whispered 'Almschli', and then, at last, 'Mozart'.

Six months later in Vienna Bruno Walter conducted the première of Mahler's Ninth Symphony.

Four years later Alma married Walter Gropius.

What happened to Miss Turner, the English Nanny, we do not know.

E. MEINHARDT

Oxford

6
Short Stories from General Practice

This quintet has general practice as its connecting strand although each tale has its own distinctive colour. There is a ghost story, a fairy story and stories about ordinary people.

The Enchantment of George: a Ghost Story from General Practice

Everyone who lived in the Greater London suburb of Harehill knew Charlie Knott. He had taught many of them at the local Grammer School where he had been head of the English Department for nearly thirty years, but he was also nationally famous as an expert on the poetry of Keats and Shelley.

At eighty-six, he was still an active member of the local literary association and his slim, slightly stooping figure was a familiar sight in the High Street. Charlie had developed a passion for computers in his retirement and was very proud of his Amstrad which he regarded as almost human, especially in the sad years after the death of his wife when his home life had become increasingly lonely.

Charlie was rarely ill. On one of his infrequent visits to the Harehill Health Centre, for some minor problem such as influenza vaccination, he happened to mention his computer to his doctor Graeme Tomlin who shared his love of poetry. Because he was the last patient and it was a quiet morning, the doctor had taken him round to the office to meet George. George came from the large family of IBM computers and had recently taken over repeat prescribing, recall for immunisation, over-eighties screening and other functions of the group practice. Tomlin had no reservations about showing Charlie how to access his own database, which contained little of importance except a few normal blood pressure recordings and

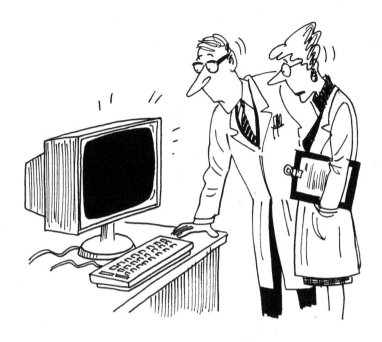

When they looked back at the screen the couplet was no longer there.

the date of his wife's death. Seeing George in action was hardly likely to cause a breach of confidentiality, he thought, as Charlie Knott would be unable to get his hands on the computer without supervision and had no knowledge of the passwords anyway.

Graeme Tomlin's friendly demonstration of George had disastrous consequences. Charlie Knott was so enthralled with the electronic wizardry that he forgot to look right as he crossed the road from the health centre and was flattened by Big Bill Brooker's council dust cart. He was killed instantly. There were plenty of witnesses who all declared that the driver had had no chance of avoiding the old man. The police breathalysed Big Bill on the spot. He was notorious in Harehill for his alcohol intake, but on this occasion he was well below the limit. He wept like a child all through the inquest, but the coroner was kind to him and returned a clear verdict of accidental death. The whole Brooker family were on Graeme

Tomlin's list. Bill's wife Josie was expecting their fifth baby in the near future, although she rarely attended for antenatal care and had missed all the usual screening tests considered essential by obstetricians and the better-educated mothers of today.

There was a memorial service for Charlie Knott in the Parish Church, which was packed. Everyone said that if *they* had to choose how to go they could not think of a better way. The vicar said that one of Harehill's institutions had passed into the service of the Almighty as the Good Lord wanted somebody to read Keats and Shelley to him, which puzzled the congregation, who considered that the spirits of original poets might lay on a divine command performance of their own.

A short while later, Graeme Tomlin was on night duty and had a call in the small hours. He was reluctant to leave his bed as he had been deeply asleep when the phone burst into life by his pillow. It was in that vitally important first hour after dropping off when waking is slow and painful and although he had managed the patient, who had called him because he thought he had appendicitis but had not, reasonably well, he still felt very much below par on the homeward journey. His route took him past the health centre. There was a green glow in the office window. 'Blast it', he thought, 'Somebody's forgotten to shut George down for the night.' He entered the building and unlocked the door to the office. George was displaying a database, the whole of which was flashing. 'That's odd,' Tomlin said out loud. 'I didn't think George behaved like that. Only cursors are supposed to flash.' He glanced at the words on the screen. It was Josie Brooker's case summary. Tomlin was about to switch the machine off when he noticed the last entry on the screen.

31 May 1988 – Fifth child – boy – normal delivery – birth weight 3.4 kg – congenital heart disease (Fallot's Tetralogy)

'That's crazy,' thought the doctor. 'I must be asleep and dreaming.' He looked at his watch. 'Yes, I thought so. It's Wednesday the 11th today.' He decided to try another file, chose Big Bill's and found another surprise. The screen recorded an incident a fortnight later than the birth of his fifth child:

10 June 1988 – Antero-septal myocardial infarction. Subsequently treated by angioplasty to left anterior descending artery

'Well, that figures', Tomlin mused. 'Bill is overweight, smokes like a chimney and takes no exercise, so I've been expecting this for some time.'

The desire to know one's own future is very strong. Sooth-sayers, signs of the zodiac, ouija boards, tarot cards and the like are nearly as powerful an influence today as occult forces were in medieval times. People laugh at superstitions, but still say 'touch wood' after the ancient belief that certain trees such as the oak and the ash have spiritual powers. They persist in avoiding the cracks in the paving stones when out shopping and look up their horoscopes each week in the columns of the newspaper. Graeme Tomlin was no fool. He regarded his work as a science with data that could be measured and he had little time for dabbling in the affairs of the supernatural. But it was one o'clock in the morning. He was tired and puzzled by George's behaviour and had almost convinced himself that the forward dates on the Brooker files were electronic mistakes. He and his family were patients on the list of his senior partner, and on impulse he keyed in a request for his own record and a few seconds later was horrified by what he saw as the last entry on his problem list.

27 June 1988 – Sudden death. Post mortem showed dissecting aneurysm of aorta

'This is getting beyond belief,' he thought and switched George off, his hands trembling a little. But he took out his notebook and wrote down carefully on a clean page what he had read about the Brookers, although he had forgotten the exact dates, and then added the sombre predictions of his own fate which, naturally enough, he remembered word for word. He went home.

Looking at his wife Margaret, who rarely stirred after twenty-five years of night calls, he wondered whether he should wake her and tell her about George, but decided not to. She was sensible and down-to-earth and he adored her, but she would have been annoyed at being disturbed and highly unlikely to be in a frame of mind to believe his extraordinary tales about a haunted computer. In fact, he had already begun to disbelieve them himself.

The following morning, Graeme Tomlin was in his shower when the strange events at his surgery during the night came back to him. He went back into the bedroom still dripping and opened his notebook. The page on which he had written down George's prophesies was empty. He wondered with slight amusement whether he was in the early stages of Alzheimer's Disease.

The days of a general practitioner in the British Health Service are long and busy. Sometimes he sees more than fifty patients in twenty-four hours and he has to concentrate on their varied problems without spending too much time in reflection about the past. It was therefore not surprising that the curious happenings of Graeme Tomlin's night on duty were soon forgotten, although he accessed George before morning surgery and checked the three bewitched files. None of them contained anything about the future. The incident was slotted into a remote corner of his subconscious mind and he threw himself back into his work as if it had never happened. But not for long.

Josie Brooker lived on the Harehill council estate. Her home was always in a state of happy squalor, with four children under the age of five crawling on the floor in the company of two huge Alsations and a tortoiseshell tabby cat who had just had a litter of six kittens. There was a haze of tobacco smoke in all the rooms. Two days before term Josie went into labour precipitately, had two contractions and pushed out a baby boy on to the kitchen floor. Granny Bradstock from next door was eighty-three and well versed in obstetrics, having had ten children herself. She tied off the cord with wool from a ball that the kittens had been playing with on the filthy carpet and cut it expertly with the knife that Big Bill had been using to peel the potatoes.

The ambulance and Claire Banks, the slightly breathless district midwife, arrived almost together to be met on the doorstep by Granny Bradstock with a toothless grin splitting her face from ear to ear and the latest Brooker in her ample arms.

The midwife retrieved Baby Brooker, who had already been christened 'Shane' after a character on television, from the clasp of her rival *accoucheuse*. Noticing that he was rather blue she gave him some oxygen before the short ambulance journey with his mother to St Elizabeth's, the local hospital. Shane remained blue despite further oxygen and the paediatrician thought that he probably had something wrong with his heart.

Graeme Tomlin first heard about the birth from Claire Banks at the antenatal clinic the next day. The precipitate labour came as no surprise, but the news of Shane's neonatal complications gave him a tight feeling in his throat that he thought with panic was probably emotionally induced angina. He rang the hospital and spoke to the paediatrician. 'Do you think it's Fallot's tetralogy?' he asked, as nonchalantly as he could, although he could feel his own heart doing its best to jump out of his chest. 'We don't think so,' replied his colleague. 'Fallots' usually presents rather later. It's probably transposition of the great vessels. Anyway, we're sending Shane up to a specialist unit in town because he'll need urgent studies to decide what's to be done.'

The birth of Shane left Graeme Tomlin decidedly uneasy. As the days went by, however, he rationalised events and gradually convinced himself that the finding of congenital heart disease was a coincidence. Moreover, he talked himself into believing that even if Big Bill should be the second of George's predictions to come true it would be no more than reasonable, as he had strong risk factors for coronary disease. He had forgotten the date of both the Brooker predictions, although his own promised end on 27 June was now once more very much on his mind. But work had to go on as before and Tomlin could not waste time in contemplation about the haunting of George. Over the next ten days the importance of the whole affair gradually faded.

Big Bill was a nifty darts player. He had even featured in a televised stage of one of the national competitions. He required at least six pints of bitter to steady his hand before a match, but despite this was a formidable opponent. On the night of 10 June he was competing for the local team at the Merry Yeoman and had just slotted his three darts into the treble twenty slot. Before the teller's cry of 'one hundred and eighty' had died away, Bill fell to the floor as if pole-axed. A senior first-aider from St John's was in the bar and he used the one opportunity for genuine cardiopulmonary resuscitation that had come his way with excellent results, so that Big Bill was delivered swiftly to the casualty department myocardially infarcted, somewhat shocked, but still alive.

Graeme Tomlin was told about the attack when he paid a final postnatal visit to Josie. He visited Bill Brooker in the ICU and spoke to the sister in charge. 'Can I see his ECG, please', he said with some trepidation. The Q waves and raised ST segments on the anterior chest leads were all too evident. Bill had, as George had said he would, blocked off his left anterior descending artery. The recovery was fairly uneventful, but although he left hospital after ten days, Bill had definite symptoms of angina and the medical team looking after him were planning further assessment with an exercise test and probably referral to a local cardiologist for angiography. Graeme had no doubt at all that that would lead to an angioplasty. His earlier determination to regard anything that happened to Big Bill as in keeping with the risk factors was totally shattered and he could think of little else except the fateful date at the end of June, now less than three weeks into the future, when he would face his own nemesis.

Tomlin was reminded of the words of Dr Samuel Johnson:

When a man knows he is to be hanged in a fortnight, it concentrates his mind wonderfully.

He felt dreadfully alone. There was nothing he could do to share his predicament. To suggest to his partners that he had prior knowledge of the medical events in the Brooker household would have made them reach for their partnership agreements to study the clause about termination for insanity. Nor could he discuss it with Margaret, who would merely have laughed and teased him about the problems of old age. Dissecting aneurysym was a pretty devastating condition, he knew, although, in his years of general practice he had never seen a case. Were there any warning signs of the catastrophe? He opened the textbook of medicine in the practice library and looked it up.

Most patients are hypertensive, he read. Well that was all right, because from a recent pension medical he knew that he was not. It was associated with degeneration of the middle coat of the aorta and could run in families. His own family was perfectly healthy. There seemed to be no way of diagnosing it before the event of rupturing into the artery wall. Pain in the chest, back and arms were the most frequent symptoms and if the patient survived the acute attack, he had little to look forward to except kidney failure and blockage of the arterial supply to the legs. All in all, a pretty nasty prognosis.

How could he get a medical opinion without revealing his name? There was only one way and that was to use the radio doctor. He rang up the local radio station at the appropriate time, said his name was Martin from Manchester and asked to speak to the doctor.

'I'm worried about my heart and circulation', he stammered, sounding just like one of the frightful people he had heard pouring out their troubles when he had in the past inadvertently tuned in to the same programme. 'Most people are these days,' came the smooth reply. 'What is it exactly that bothers you?' 'I think I have an aneurysm.' There was a shocked silence. At least that's taken the wind out of his sails, Graeme thought to himself with a smile. It was unheard of for this particular media medic to be short of words. 'Er . . . have you felt a lump in your tummy?' 'No – it's what is called a dissecting aneurysm I'm concerned about.' 'Oh yes, that happens in the chest to the main artery we call the aorta as it rises up from the heart. Why do you think you've got that?' 'I get pains in the chest and back. Is there any way you can tell before the thing bursts?' 'Well now look, Martin from Manchester. Dissecting aneurysm is very rare and I doubt if you've got one from what you tell me. All the same I think it might be a good idea for you to go down and see your doctor about it in the next few days.' There followed much gratuitous reassurance and nebulous waffle, and Martin alias Graeme was bidden farewell. All these radio consultations end in the same way, Graeme thought gloomily as he hung up. Fat lot of use those conceited idiots in the studio were, considering the massive amount they were paid.

What should he do now? Graeme Tomlin had a scornful disregard for the 'executive medical' carried out in private clinics, but desperate situations call for desperate measures. He made a surreptitious appointment in the city on his half-day, told his wife that he had to pick up a book from the BMA library and presented himself for the comprehensive check-up that he knew was a total waste of time and money but which would at least be confidential. No, he declared firmly when asked, he did not want his own doctor even to know he had attended, let alone be sent a report of the findings. They were to be for his eyes only.

The marathon overhaul was completely normal. His chest X-ray, ECG, blood chemistry and clinical findings were without exception totally satisfactory and he received a typically flattering letter from the doctor who saw him, going over all the uneventful minutiae of his medical history, telling him that he was fitter than a man half his age and hoping that he would return for another examination in a year's time. 'A chance,' he muttered to himself, 'Would be a fine thing!'

Inevitably, Tomlin experienced chest pains and backache in the days ahead. He felt his radial and femoral pulses every few minutes to make sure that they had not begun to diminish, sweated at every palpitation and became so snappy and withdrawn that his colleagues and staff wondered what was wrong. To his dismay, Big Bill did progress to an angioplasty and rather against the odds, his little son Shane was found to have the classical four abnormalities of Fallot's tetralogy. By now the doctor's seventeen days grace after Bill Brooker's coronary had dwindled to three.

George did not help. He remained stubbornly mute on the fortune-telling although the Brooker files were appended appropriately by the office staff. There seemed to be nothing left to do. Papers in order, debts paid, Dr Tomlin awaited his fate with courage and resignation. He wondered at what time of the day the end would come. Would it be during morning surgery or at coffee afterwards? He hoped he would not collapse at the wheel and run into anyone else in the street. On the night of 26 June, after lying awake for several hours, he eventually fell into troubled slumber. His last conscious thought was that death in his sleep would save a lot of trouble.

The morning of 27 June dawned bright and full of birdsong as even in Britain it is inclined to do at this time of the year. Graeme Tomlin left for the health centre after giving Margaret an extra long hug. He did not have long to await his fearsome outcome. His youngest partner Jim Peck was the only other doctor in the common-room when he went in with his post.

'I didn't know you had a vasectomy in your thirties', he said looking up with a cheeky grin. 'What do you mean', said Tomlin, feeling a flush spreading up to the roots of his hair. 'I had to go out early this morning to a chap who collapsed and died with chest and back pain. I'll have to let the coroner know later, although I expect it was a coronary. He's a new patient, just registered with me. Almost your namesake actually, but he spells his name Graham Tomlins. George put up your file by mistake – sorry!' 'It was a dissecting aneurysm', murmured Tomlin almost to himself. 'Well, we're not all psychic', said his young colleague with a sarcastic smirk. 'Lesser mortals like me will have to wait for the PM.' But of course, it was.

Graeme Tomlin was in the health centre office a month later when the computer operator, Penny Blake, called him over to have a look at George. 'This is a bit odd', she said. 'I've just put up the file of that nice old chap Charlie Knott you brought in here just before he was killed. I know the doctors like to keep a print-out of the files of patients who have died or left the list. Someone's been mucking about. Look, there's an entry that's flashing and George never does that. What does it mean, anyway?'

Tomlin looked at the screen. In the middle of the file were two lines of poetry.

The soul of Adonais like a star
Beacons from the abode where the Eternal are

'It's Shelley', he said. 'Writing about John Keats. I expect old Charlie keyed it in himself. He was an expert on both of them.' 'For a second, doctor, I thought you were being serious', retorted Penny casting him a withering look. 'I was', said Tomlin eagerly, 'Print it out.' But George would not. Only the medical data on Charlie Knott's file appeared on the paper, and when they looked back at the screen, the couplet was no longer there.

JOHN WOODWARD

Sidcup

Prentice Finch

Market Middleford is a sleepy little town so exactly in the centre of England that parents there with young children often complain about the distance to the coast. It may have wondered what it had done to deserve Prentice Finch. His name caused despair in the heart of every doctor in the Market Middleford Group Practice. The best way to describe him would be to say that he had all the worst faults of Steptoe Senior and Alf Garnett with none of their charisma. Finch was seventy-eight at the time this story ends. He had once been a postman, but had not worked for thirty years, having retired early because of his health. The diagnosis then had been 'angina', but there was precious little to show for it in his medical records.

How Prentice Finch obtained his first name was a matter of some conjecture. It was said that his father, Albert, who had been a much-respected carpenter in the town, had been grateful to his employer to whom he had been apprenticed for three years and christened his son with a shortened version of the word apprentice. It sounded improbable but that was the reason old Finch always gave when asked. It could also be claimed that Jennie Prentice, an illicit flame from a nearby village who, unknown to Albert's wife, consumed him on occasions, had something to do with it.

There were many medical events in the history of Prentice Finch. He was reputed to have had a heart attack at the age of sixty-one, although the cardiographic and biochemical evidence for this illness was equivocal. His notes recorded that he was a chronic bronchitic but his early morning cough, although lusty enough to disturb neighbours in the terrace where he lived as far as four doors away in either direction, was rarely accompanied by objective clinical signs of airways obstruction. It was his own distinctive and quite irresistible mating call. Not that Finch had actually mated for twenty years. Even then it had been a fairly perfunctory performance, according to his wife Mary, several years younger, who had grown up in Kilkenny and used Dr Ian Jones, her GP, as a father confessor on occasions and to whom she bared her soul. No, Prentice produced his lusty stag-like bellow as a reminder to Mary that in his frailty he needed the constant and undivided *domestic* attention of a mate, promised him more than fifty years earlier in Middleford's Catholic Church.

Prentice Finch was also diabetic, supposed to be following a diet which had been carefully transcribed for him by the dietician in the diabetic clinic at Middleton Hospital. He followed all her instructions, and then supplemented his intake freely with doughnuts, chocolate, ginger biscuits and in an emergency if Mary forgot to replenish his supplies of these favoured victuals, bread and strawberry jam. In the last five years he had also developed diverticulitis, osteoarthritis of the hips, nodular prurigo of the shins (self-induced by scratching) and trigeminal neuralgia to add to the summary list in his records.

Despite constant admonitions from his doctor Finch was an inveterate smoker. The ceiling in the lounge of his minute Victorian house in Osborne Terrace was coloured deep brown with smoke. The carpet was peppered with holes from falling ash. Those visiting him had some difficulty in discerning his portly form, sitting immovably in the battered fireside chair which he defended fiercely as his own exclusive territory, because of the evil-smelling haze which hung over the room.

Finch's list of medication was impressive. He took beta-blockers for his angina, which surprisingly had few adverse effects on his respiratory problems; the heart was also boosted by digoxin and diuretics, long-acting nitrates and aminophylline. Added to these were pain-killers for his arthritis and neuralgia, vitamins, sleeping tablets and antihistamines for his itchy skin. Finch's most treasured possession of all, however, was an oxygen set which stood cylindrical and reassuring, but totally unnecessary, beside his favourite chair. Ian Jones had prescribed it in a moment of weakness and for Prentice it was the most conspicuous symbol he possessed of the legitimacy of his sick role. In the company of visitors, he frequently reached out for the life-giving mask taking convulsive gasps through its transparent tubing, but few of his startled friends ever noticed that he rarely turned on the cylinder as he did so.

Yet despite his apparent dependence on drugs and avowed inability to attend the Middleford surgery because of his heart, Finch was by no means confined to his house. He regularly walked across the local recreation ground supported by a walking stick provided by the Social Services to visit the Cock and Bull in Middleford High Street for his pint drawn from the wood. Here he would complain bitterly to the landlord, or anyone else who would listen, about the incompetence of his doctor, the stupidity of Mary and the hopelessness of those who paid out his pension in the Post Office. He could also be heard on long summer Saturdays shouting obscenities at the Middleford batsmen from under the thick canopy of the horse chestnuts which ringed the cricket ground behind the Catholic Church.

Now and then, Prentice Finch managed to persuade one of the doctors in the practice that he was genuinely ill. It was usually when one of the young trainees was on duty, someone who would be unacquainted with his dramatic skills, and he could be alarmingly convincing. These episodes usually took the form of chest pain. Finch knew all the symptoms of myocardial infarction right down to such details as the exact site in the left arm to which the pain was referred and he had been admitted on several occasions to the intensive care unit of Middleford Hospital, where the medical registrar was as befuddled as the family doctors about his true condition.

On one of these admissions, Finch actually did have a heart attack – at least, his heart stopped beating. No cardiographic changes subsequently developed, but it must have been a bout of ventricular fibrillation. It was after he had been moved to the ordinary ward, because as usual nothing had come to light in intensive care from the standard battery of tests. To the dismay of everyone who knew him at the surgery, in Osborne Terrace or in the Cock and Bull, an alert staff nurse happened to notice that he had turned blue and was not breathing. In the ward at the same time was a keen young house physician, who had thrown himself onto Finch's chest in a long dive worthy of any international scrum half feeding his stand off and pummelled the miserable man's myocardium back into life.

It was this unfortunate resuscitation which had taken Mary in despair to Dr Jones. 'I know I'm wicked, father,' she had wept (Ian had grown used to being confused with Patrick Murphy, the Catholic Priest in Middleford, and indeed in this regular confessional their roles were often blurred). 'I pray about it every day and I tell Father Murphy at confession and ask the Good Lord to forgive me, but I hope he dies. I do, doctor, I hope he dies and does it soon. And doctor, if he does die, I pray to God that he dies when he's out somewhere, because if he dies at home I shall have to call the doctor and then he'll recover.' 'Don't worry, Mary,' Ian had said soothingly. 'I don't think God blames you for how you feel. I expect He knows what you have to put up with.' 'I do that,' Mary had confided, 'look at what he did yesterday morning'. And she had pulled up her sleeve to show him a great bruise around the upper part of her arm where Prentice had grabbed her and shaken her because she had not come at once with his cough medicine when his hoarse pre-breakfast bark had shattered the calm of Osborne Terrace. Ian Jones could well believe it. He had felt the old man's fury too, especially during one memorable home visit when he had told the troublesome patient that there was really no reason why he should not come down to see him in surgery in view of the fact that he regularly visited the Post Office, which was even further along the road than the surgery. Prentice had reached for his walking stick and with a wide, swift, unavoidable sweep had given Ian a severe blow behind his left ear. The other partners had suggested that Prentice Finch should be struck off the list, but Jones had felt sorry for Mary Finch and had refused to retaliate in this way, although he had had good cause to do so.

Prentice Finch was the sworn enemy of all the children in

Osborne Terrace. Any ball that happened to land in his tiny garden was promptly cut in half and hurled back across the fence, to the accompaniment of a stream of foul oaths. Young people fled from him as he strode across the street waving his terrible stick and he could spit with legendary accuracy, so he was a formidable adversary. It was never proved, but there was much circumstantial evidence to link him with the drowning of a kitten belonging to Clare and Timothy Jarvis, the six-year-old twins who lived next door. It had strayed across onto his land and everyone in the terrace suspected him of throwing it into his water butt and then leaving it sodden and lifeless on the Jarvis's doorstep. Not a nice man, Prentice Finch.

To everything, wrote the authors of the Book of Ecclesiastes, there is a time to be born and a time to die. It seemed on a frosty Monday morning in February a few years ago as if the time for the latter had at last arrived for Prentice Finch. 'Can you come quickly, doctor.' Mary, in a state of some agitation, was calling from the Jarvis's as she had no telephone. 'Prentice really is ill this time. I think it's his heart.' Ian asked his receptionist to tell the remaining patients waiting to see him that he had been summoned to an emergency and left at once. Playing wolf was a dangerous game, he thought grimly to himself as he swept down the High Street, but every situation had to be assessed before it could be dismissed as a triviality. This was part of what made general practice such a fascinating and infuriating job.

It was obvious that the visit was different from normal. Mary was waiting anxiously for him in the doorway. This had never happened before. All Prentice's previous cries for help had obviously been much less alarming to her. Ian Jones thanked his stars that he had not left it until the end of surgery. Finch was lying in bed in the front room upstairs. His face was pale and slightly blue and he was in considerable pain. Jones felt for his pulse – thready and fast, at about 120. His blood pressure was almost unrecordable, the sphygmomanometer suggested 70 over 50, but it was hard to hear anything at Prentice's elbow as the cuff deflated. The heart sounds were so faint that they too were hardly audible, but at least Finch's lung bases sounded clear. As yet there were no definite signs of failure. Jones injected 5 mg of diamorphine slowly into a vein, although it was not easy to find one. Gradually, Finch's expression of terror faded – terror of death, perhaps, or of more pain, or just panic and consternation about what was going to happen to him. Fear was the worst symptom of all, though Jones with his hand on Finch's pulse, and morphine, which spread calm over it like the stillness of a lake in the evening, remained one of the best of all the drugs available to doctors.

Prentice Finch was probably going to die. For the moment though, the diamorphine had done its work and he was much more comfortable. Ian Jones went downstairs with Mary. 'What would you like me to do?' he asked her gently. 'We could get him into hospital, if you like, but I think he is very ill and he's probably going to die whatever we decide.' 'If that's the case, I'd rather he stayed at home,' said Mary, and Jones admired her pluck and faithfulness despite the hard time her cantankerous husband had given her for all their long married life. He remembered what she had said to him after Prentice's cardiac arrest in Middleford Hospital.

Upstairs, Prentice had sunk into sleep. Ian checked his pulse and blood pressure again before he left. The pressure had come up to 100 over 70 and his pulse was stable without ex-trasystoles; his colour had also improved slightly. 'I'll call back again in a couple of hours and do an ECG,' he said. Ian Jones was proud of the practice ECG machine. It had cost the partnership a lot of money and he liked using it even though it would make little difference to the management of Prentice Finch.

When Ian Jones returned, Prentice was still asleep and there was no sign of deterioration in his condition. The dangerous first hour had passed, but Jones still was not sanguine about the outcome. He was an old man, after all, and even though many of his past illnesses had been imaginary the years had taken their toll. The ECG was quite definite. It showed a large anterior infarct with reciprocal changes in the posterior leads denoting the loss of a considerable amount of cardiac muscle.

'Do you think we should get Father Patrick?' asked Mary. 'Of course, if you would like to'. Jones replied, 'but I don't think the end is imminent. I'll look back again this evening. Are you sure you can still manage?' Mary nodded her assent.

On the third visit, Jones could see that there had been a change. Prentice was more short of breath and there were crepitations at both pulmonary bases. Also, his heart showed a triple rhythm – clear evidence that he was in cardiac failure. As he watched by the bed, his hand on the patient's wrist, Prentice's pulse began to throw off runs of heart block, a slow ventricular rate of about 40 beats a minute. Prentice was no longer conscious.

'Perhaps it's time for Father Murphy now,' he told Mary downstairs. 'I'll give him an injection of diuretics to help his breathing.' Patrick duly arrived and began to administer the last rites. There was a great dignity about the scene and Ian remembered Elgar's setting of the Dream of Gerontius, a work which always affected him greatly. The steady voice of the priest on a single note commending the dying man to his maker – go forth upon thy journey, Christian Soul, go in the name of God . . .

Prentice Finch always was a difficult man. Irascible and violent, selfish and capricious, his soul was in no mood to do as it was told. As soon as Patrick started to pray, Finch began to recover. His pulse steadied to sinus rhythm at 76. His blood pressure rose to 130 over 80. He opened his eyes and when he saw Patrick, he swore. 'Bugger off,' he muttered. 'Did she call you? I ain't dead yet, blast you'. Father Murphy withdrew in some confusion, and Ian had to pacify him over a cup of tea downstairs. Patrick took sometime to forgive the doctor for getting it wrong, but when the two men met in Middleford Hospital a few weeks later, Ian pointed out that Finch had been confusing the whole medical community for most of his life, so it was not surprising that he should do the same to the priesthood. 'And the Good Lord too,' said Father Murphy with a grin. 'I expect He was getting ready a few surprises for the old devil!'

Despite the extent of Prentice Finch's myocardial infarct, he made a complete recovery. Within three weeks he was spitting at the children again and swiping at them with his stick. He was furious with Mary for calling the priest to give him the last rites. He did not share his wife's Catholic faith and thought that all priests were a bunch of crooks, not to be trusted with anything, least of all the safe passage of his soul. But then, of course, he did not really believe in his soul either.

Mary's life became a succession of abuses, accusations and assaults. Prentice worked out in the faulty synapses of his arteriosclerotic brain that she had in some way been in league with the doctor and the priest in a plot to do away with him. He refused to take any more tablets, which actually did not matter at all because he did not need them. He made Mary taste everything she cooked in the house in case he was being poisoned and on his daily perambulations across the recreation ground he would shout out his suspicions at passers-by: 'She's trying to kill me, you know,' he would yell, 'and that bloody doctor too. They're all in it together'. He became unbearable in the Cock and Bull and the landlord was furious because the bar emptied as soon as Finch's wild eyes appeared on the threshold. 'He ought to be put away', he said, and the cry was echoed around Market Middleford: 'He ought to be put away. Why don't they do something?'

The social worker was alerted and visited the Finch household, but was smitten on the nose with Prentice's walking stick. He retired to discuss the matter with his team leader. They held a case conference, but decided after three hours of fruitless discussion that they were not authorised to do anything so they refused to play any further part in the proceedings. The community psychiatric nurse interviewed him warily from a safe distance across the room, but no distance in the house was safe from Prentice's other weapon and he left swiftly, wiping tobacco-stained spittle from his eye. The consultant psychogeriatrician arrived on one of Prentice's good days. The old codger was charm itself and talked at length about the war and his garden and how the terrace had changed in the last few years and would the kind doctor like a cup of tea and when would he be calling again? With seventy-three other elderly patients waiting for his opinion, it is not surprising that the consultant breathed a sigh of relief and crossed Prentice Finch off his list of patients needing urgent admission.

'I shall live for years,' gloated Finch to Mary. 'You can't put me away. The social worker bloke can't put me away nor that bloody nurse. The consultant thought I was all right and he should know. I'm off to the pub. If you ain't got me lunch ready when I get back I'll beat the hell out of you so hard that you won't be able to go to your confessions with that sod Murphy'. And as he stomped off to the Cock and Bull he turned and threw back a final defiance. 'You can't kill me. The doctor can't kill me. Even that priest and his God can't kill me. I'll outlive all you buggers, just see if I don't!'

God, however, though He may have appeared to have been somewhat deceived by Prentice Finch's escape from the last rites, is not mocked. Our indestructible anti-hero returned from his pint in the empty bar with the glowering landlord and was about to enter his house when a rubber ball bounced into the little square front garden. He turned in fury to see who had thrown it. Just at that minute a slate on his roof, loosened by the October gales, slid smoothly over the gutter and dropped vertically. Its fall was arrested by the old man's head, which it shattered as an egg shatters on the side of a saucepan. Prentice never felt a thing. He collapsed in a sitting posture onto a large flower pot beside the front door, indisputably dead.

The residents of Osborne Terrace gathered in wonder in the street to witness the macabre sight until someone covered the body with a blanket and called the police. Mary asked Father Patrick to come and say a prayer and although he looked suspiciously at Prentice's remains as if he thought that they might come to life again, he obliged and at least Mary felt that the old chap for whom she bore no malice had started on his journey with a blessing. There was an inquest, of course. It could only return a verdict of accidental death, but neither Mary nor Father Patrick were so sure that providence had no part in it.

Although Father Murphy could not quite bring himself to allow Prentice to lie at rest in the graveyard of his church, he did agree to Mary's request for a small tablet in a corner of the garden. The inscription it bore was short and apt. *In memory of Prentice Finch*, it said simply, and then there was a quotation from the First Book of Samuel – *a man after his own heart*.

JOHN WOODWARD

Sidcup

Mary Ella and the Slipper: a Modern Fairy Tale

M iss Mary Ella Hinge described herself as elderly spinster and maiden aunt. In reality, as she approached her sixtieth birthday, she had the looks and vigour of youthful middle-age. But she was unmarried and likely to remain so.

In three months she was to retire from her part-time job at the local supermarket; several others were leaving at the same time, and a dinner dance had been arranged to celebrate the occasion. Mary had spent some weeks deciding on what to wear; she rarely socialised and intended to make the evening 'a right good do!' The outfit she eventually bought was a flattering shade of royal blue, complemented by a beautiful pair of sequinned high-heeled shoes, which would show off her trim ankles to perfection. They might even draw an admiring glance from Mr Charm, her supervisor, who also was retiring.

Mary Ella had been working for only five years: previously she had looked after her ailing mother and handicapped father. Her two sisters, being married, had left the bulk of the caring to Mary. When her parents died, she was able to enjoy her freedom until her eldest sister Gladys, who was now a widow, adopted the sick role which had for so long belonged to their mother.

Gladys was an habitual attender at my surgery. Her status at the practice was demonstrated by the fact that an envelope had recently been constructed to house a second set of notes. In the last few months she had taken to calling me out on home visits and was collecting a fair number of pills and potions in her jumbo-sized drug cabinet, not all of them prescribed. Many of her problems stemmed from her size, for which Gladys blamed her glands and I blamed her mouth. Nineteen stone and rising, she was secretly envious of her sister's slim figure and used her as a general dogsbody for shopping and cleaning, although their homes were two miles apart.

The dream blue outfit was less than well received by Gladys. 'I wouldn't be seen dead in that!' Mary Ella knew better than to answer back to her sister, the dress being several sizes too small for Gladys. The shoes were similarly dismissed as 'too frivolous for her age.'

The youngest sister, Celia, appeared to be the happiest of the family. Her husband kept her in some luxury and tolerated her thirty cigarettes-a-day habit. Though he was rarely at home due to work and social commitments, he was the proud father of three children and grandfather to five. Mary Ella was much thought of by these offspring. She was invariably available for baby-sitting duties; after all, she never went out.

Six weeks before the big day, Gladys was already anticipating the time after which her sister would be exclusively hers for the washing and nursing of her frail form. For a few days, Mary had noticed that her ankles were swelling. Then she seemed to become unusually tired after carrying the shopping home. One night she woke up breathless. She shrugged off the symptoms as a sign of age and they went unnoticed by her nearest and dearest. It was hard to ignore the evidence that presented one evening. The sequinned shoes, so delicate, so beautiful, would no longer fit her expanding feet. She mentioned the matter to Gladys, who was quick to point out that everyone's feet swelled at the end of the day, and what did she expect at her age anyway. The offending shoes had always been inappropriate and Gladys would be happy to lend a pair of hers for the occasion, if Mary still insisted on wasting her time on such frivolity.

The predicament of her sister had affected Gladys; it reminded her of the water retention that had plagued her intermittently for years, and the memory precipitated one of her attacks. She felt ill and feeble. When Mary called with the shopping the next morning, she was greeted by the news that the doctor had been summoned. Mary was too breathless to register the information as she half-collapsed into a chair, too exhausted to answer my ring. To Gladys's chagrin, I was more interested in the state of the stricken Mary than in her sister's condition. Mary rarely attended the surgery and she was a stranger to me. I asked her to lie down, and examined her thoroughly; I knew I would discover more pathology in this patient than in Gladys's mighty medical tomes. By the time I had finished, Mary was feeling a little better, and I asked her to come down to the surgery later that day for some tests.

In a few days the water pills that I had prescribed had worked wonders for both Mary's moral and her feet. As Mary explained to Celia, the diagnosis was mild heart failure due to high blood pressure. Celia found this highly amusing. 'The doctors said that smoking would kill me', she said. 'My heart's in fine condition, and look at you. No vices, no worries and no children, but you're the one with the health problems!'

I had said it would be difficult to pin down Mary's hypertension to any particular cause, but that stress might be playing a part in the condition. Without being fully aware of the family dynamics, I was glad that Mary would soon be retiring, as I thought that the extra outside work might be contributing to the situation. Mary was thankful to be feeling better. In her eyes I had certainly waved some magic wand and she hesitated to contradict me; she realised that the stress was mainly due to her sisters' attitudes and particularly to Gladys's constant demand for attention. Her job was a lifeline to the outside world, and she did not know how she was going to cope without it.

At last the great day dawned; the dress was freshly pressed and the shoes were the snuggest of fits. In the afternoon Mary was sitting with her feet up and relaxing when the phone rang. It was Gladys. 'Oh Mary', she cried, 'I'm so poorly. Will you come round and see me at once.' The line went dead. Mary pulled on her coat and for once in her life called a taxi. She was filled with an awful sense of foreboding. To her surprise her sister looked much as usual; perhaps a little paler but certainly no frailer. Moreover, there were no new symptoms to account for the urgent call. It soon transpired that Gladys was feeling lonely and weak, with an inability to cope with her ordinary tasks. She would not get out of her bed to go to the toilet; she could not possibly manage to make a drink for herself; in short, she wanted Mary Ella to spend the night with her until she felt stronger. Mary was flabbergasted. It was obvious that Gladys was trying to prevent the evening's entertainment. Mary called Celia. There was no help forthcoming from that quarter. Celia was much too busy. In desperation, Mary called the surgery and asked to speak to me. Luckily, I was available, and was as annoyed as ever with Gladys's gambits. 'There is nothing wrong with your sister, Miss Hinge. Certainly nothing that makes it dangerous to leave her alone tonight. You go out and enjoy yourself and I'll call round tomorrow.' For the first time in her life, Mary found the courage to say no to her sister and to act on my words. 'Gladys, I'm going out. I'll see you later. I should be back around midnight.'

It was a wonderful evening. Mary forgot the time as she waltzed and foxtrotted away the hours, and most of her dances were with Mr Charm, who was most attentive. He had told Mary how wonderful she looked at the beginning of the evening, and seemed unable to keep his eyes off her. It was well known that he had been a widower for some years and had been reluctant to retire to an empty house. Mary was just a little bit tipsy and was picturing herself as a companion in that empty house when the clock struck midnight. In horror she remembered her poorly sister. 'I've got to go', she murmured. She had already arranged for a taxi to collect her and hurried to the exit. Her feet had become slightly swollen with the heat and dancing. In order to walk properly, she was forced to remove her sequinned shoes. In her haste she dropped one as she left.

Of course, Gladys, though tearful, was no worse, but Mary decided to stay a day or two with her. On the second day she had a visitor. Mr Charm had called. He had spent the previous twenty-four hours tracking her down; the other women at work had known about her two sisters. He had called at Celia's first, and was glad to find no trace of Mary in the smoke-filled rooms.

'I came to return this', he smiled, handing her the missing shoe, which fitted her perfectly once more. 'Would you like to come to dinner with me tonight?'

It would be satisfying to report that they all lived happily ever after. I was happy with my patient's recovery and managed to persuade a disappointed Gladys to go into a home with round-the-clock attention. I have no magic to induce Celia to stop smoking and she continues to puff and wheeze her days away. And Mary Ella and her husband have no complaints.

JILL THISTLETHWAITE

Luddendon

Hypertension

White-haired Dr Wilfred Peckham looked up wearily from the notes before him, pressed a button on his intercom and sat back. He was quiet. His receptionist knew his ways and a beep on her intercom meant that he was ready for the next patient. 'There we are, Mr Herbert. Doctor will see you now.'

The man in question sprang to his feet and made for the surgery door. He had a spring in his step, a twinkle in his eye and a rose in his buttonhole. He stopped on the threshold: 'Dr Peckham?' The older man looked at the younger and made a sign that he should sit in the chair opposite his desk, then his head dipped as he made a series of notes. Had Tony Herbert seen what was written he might have been interested to know that it was nothing more than a shopping list of things needing to be bought before the day was out – for Dr Peckham lived alone.

'What d'you want?' he asked suddenly. 'You wanted to see me.' 'Ah yes – wait just a moment, would you?' he pressed his buzzer. 'Yes, doctor?' said a metallic female voice. 'I have Mr Herbert in here. Didn't we have some kind of communication about him?' Tony Herbert shifted in his chair. He was well-built and no longer young, upwardly thrusting, or even mobile. He was a man at the top with all the cares and responsibilities of a king who rules over a precariously balanced economy. Wilfred Peckham had been the family's doctor for many years. Tony had always been irritated by his slowness and apparent indifference to what was happening. In Tony's line of business, the papers would have been on his desk and he would have been briefed – yes, briefed – before any client so much as came near him.

Dr Peckham's lack of power was infuriating: he had it in him to be so much more efficient. In his shoes, Tony would have fired that receptionist years ago and replaced her with someone brighter; someone familiar with filing and computers and new technology. It was all the more annoying because Tony Herbert could feel himself becoming annoyed about the whole thing – quite unreasonably so – and Peckham was harmless enough. It would do no good to be cross with him; not when he had not done anything – not a damned thing.

There was a quick tap at the door and the receptionist handed a letter to the doctor. 'Ah yes – this is it. Now then, Tony, you went for an insurance medical recently.' 'That's right.' 'Well – you had a slightly elevated blood pressure and they want me to take three more readings.' 'Why, for heaven's sake? I was fit enough there.' 'Did the doctor tell you that?' 'Not in as many words – no.' 'He shouldn't have said a word, you know. He's meant to say nothing.' 'That's a bit daft, isn't it; I mean to say . . .' 'Slip off your jacket and just go and sit in that chair over their.' Dr Peckham had a way of cutting across the bows of even the biggest steamship.

Tony Herbert felt even more angry for a moment, but he complied – took off his jacket, rolled up his sleeve and did as he was told. The cuff was applied and the doctor pumped it up. Tony had never liked that sensation when the beating and thumping began in his arm. He hated it; dreaded it. It was one of the things he feared most. 'What can you hear, doctor?' he tried a cheerful line of chat. 'Quiet now! I'm listening.' Tony felt abashed. The pressure was released and he looked at the doctor expectantly: 'Well?' 'I'm afraid I'm paid the princely sum of ten pounds fifty to provide three readings, Tony. I am not allowed to say anything to you as to the result.' 'But that's ridiculous!' 'That's as may be, my boy, but I am but a servant to the insurance company that has asked me to do this for them. I have to do this for them, not for you – even though you are employing them to cover your life – it is life, isn't it?' Tony nodded.

The next reading was even higher than the first but Dr Peckham, poker-faced as ever, gave no indication that this was so. Instead, he chatted about this and that until he was interrupted by Tony. 'What is that thumping in my arm, doctor?' 'Those thumpings, as you call them, are your arterial walls slapping their sides together. They produce a noise that was first described by a Russian called Korotkov – in 1905.' 'That's quite normal then?' 'Oh yes – quite normal.' There was genuine reassurance there. Tony felt himself beginning to relax. 'Well ⌐that's it then?' 'Yes – all done now. You may go.' 'And you can't say what the result is?' 'It is not for me to say anything, my boy. The medical chaps at the company are the ones who decide; they have columns of figures and they compare the results with them and assess the risk.' 'But surely – you *know* me?' 'Oh my goodness me – of course I do. But this is an insurance company. They don't know you. They have to have some way of assessing the risk, don't they?' 'You think I'm a risk then?' 'I didn't say that. The word "risk" is no more than just a word.' 'So – I'm alright then?' 'For the purposes of this meeting – yes; you are alright.' 'Good.' Tony Herbert stood up. 'I'll send these results to the company, you see – and then they'll write to you.' 'Thanks.'

Wilfred Peckham sat back at his desk as the younger man left and looked at the figures he had written down. The systolic had never come below a hundred and sixty and had been as high as two hundred – and the diastolic had never gone below a hundred and five. He folded the form and put it in its designated envelope before pressing his intercom buzzer for the next patient. 'Enid?' He broke his usual silence. 'Yes, doctor?' 'That fellow, Herbert . . .' 'Yes, doctor?' 'Make a note about him for me, would you?' 'Yes, doctor.' 'Just a short note, y'know – to the effect that I ought to have him back.' 'Yes, doctor.' '. . . and Enid?' 'Yes, doctor?' 'What's for supper tonight?'

It was about a week later that Tony Herbert heard from his insurance broker to the effect that he had been deferred until his blood pressure was attended to. He felt confused, upset – and betrayed. Dr Peckham had let him down in a big way by not coming clean over the blood pressure issue. He would have something to say alright – oh yes. Feathers would fly if he had anything to do with it. He fumed quietly over the problem as he drove home to his wife that evening.

'. . . he told me; I heard him say quite distinctly that there was nothing to worry about.' 'If that's what he said, then you haven't got to worry, darling.' His wife had always had a soothing influence on him. She had to have. He needed a soft landing at the end of a hard day where high-flying meant turbulence and buffeting of all kinds – and the need to stay in control at all times. '. . . but he said . . .' Tony Herbert's voice faded away to a mumble. 'Why don't you get changed into something more comfortable? If you've got blood pressure, then count yourself lucky it's been found while you're still young enough.' 'But I've always been perfectly well. It's ridiculous to think that a mere blood pressure machine can tell anything.' 'As it happens, Dr Peckham's receptionist was on the telephone only this morning.' 'Why didn't you say?' 'I was waiting for you to calm down.' 'So – what happens now?' 'You've got to see him in the morning.' 'Oh yes – and what if I'd had an appointment, eh?' 'You'd have had to cancel it, wouldn't you, darling? After all – health comes first.'

The following morning he was at the surgery exactly at a quarter past nine. He had only a five-minute wait this time; the buzzer sounded and he was on his feet and through the door even before the light went out. He sat down opposite the doctor and glared at him. The doctor looked up and returned the baleful stare. 'I thought you said I was alright and that there was nothing to worry about?' 'No man can serve two masters, Tony. My task was that of serving the company you applied to for insurance. That – was last time. Now – I am free to attend to you.' 'But you lied to me, doctor.' Tony narrowed his eyes. 'It may have appeared as a lie to you, my boy, but it was never intended as such. You have to face the fact that you're going to have to learn to calm down a bit. You really can't afford to carry on like this, you know.' 'Why not?' 'Because you'll get something happening to you . . .' 'Like what?' 'Oh – it could be a number of things. I really wouldn't want to worry you with the details.' 'Try me, doctor.' 'You have to understand, Tony, that insurance is a gamble, a game of chance, if you will; where you, the player, are given the comfortable feeling that you may be about to beat the man who keeps the table. In this case, it hasn't worked out.' 'I acted in good faith. I always act in good faith.' Tony could feel himself becoming annoyed again. 'I wasn't suggesting for a moment that you didn't. But you have to understand that this is a blessing in disguise.'

'It's a blot on my record.' 'Nonsense! In ten years time you'll say that you were glad it was found now and not then.' 'I've always been efficient, doctor. If I worked here I'd make things a lot more efficient.' 'And I'd suffer with high blood pressure on the strength of it, I expect! No Tony – you can't escape the fact that you have a problem with your blood pressure and you'll have to have it monitored for a bit until I'm convinced that it really is up.' 'What? No pills? No wonder-drugs?' 'Nope. We wait. I'd like you to buy a blood pressure machine.' 'Oh come off it, doc. You're having me on.' 'I was never more serious. Here's the address of a supplier – and don't get an electronic one. They're not as accurate as the others.' Tony Herbert puffed out his cheeks and then exhaled gently. 'You say no pills?' There was a nod from the white-headed sage. '. . . OK then. How much is a BP machine?' 'Not very much. You'll soon learn how to take your own blood pressure, and that nice wife of yours will help you if there are any problems. Wasn't she a nurse?' 'Yes but . . .' 'Good. Then that's it for now. Come back and see me again in a month.'

It was odd the way the old boy could manipulate a conversation so neatly. He could not have been in there for more than five minutes; he had wanted to say so many things, and had – in fact – managed to say nothing. And he was still not insured, either. That evening, after supper, he spoke to his wife: 'I've got to buy a BP machine.' 'Yes, darling.' 'What d'you mean 'yes, darling' like that?' 'You mustn't be cross, but I already have.' 'Ah . . .' 'The doctor gave me a ring.' 'You mean – he actually rang you?' Tony could hardly believe his ears. 'Yes – why not? He obviously cares, darling.' 'He gave me the impression that he couldn't give a toss.' 'You can hardly blame him. You don't exactly encourage compassion.' 'What d'you mean by that?' 'Like I said darling – I think you must have frightened him a bit.' 'Ha! Me frighten him? Nonsense! More like the other way round.' '. . . he asked if I could help him.' 'Eh?' Tony blinked. '. . . with the blood pressure machine; he felt that he was speaking to thin air; that you might not have heard what he was saying.' 'I heard every word.' 'When do you have to go back there?' 'Oh – I don't know about that. I've only just been, haven't I?' 'Well – it's a month, darling.' 'I wonder who looks after doctors when they go wrong?' His wife smiled cheerfully: 'No-one very much.' 'You'd better do the business. Everything has to be recorded.' 'Alright, darling. Roll up your sleeve.'

In the days that followed, an interesting thing happened. Tony's blood pressure began to settle, and after two weeks the high figures recorded for the insurance medical were now history. His interest was unbounded and he could not wait to get back to Wilfred Peckham to tell him what was happening. It was most odd – and there was no reason for the drop in BP to account for it. Business was as busy as ever and there were still the everyday wheels and deals that he wheeled and dealt, with never so much as a passing thought for his blood pressure.

His wife took his blood pressure twice a day and recorded scores that hovered around the one-twenty/sixty mark. In addition, Tony reported that he had never felt better. And two weeks later . . .

'I can't tell you what a wonderful little gadget this thing is, Dr Peckham. My wife has measured my blood pressure twice a day and it's come right down. I've never felt better.' 'Splendid! You say your wife has taken the blood pressure?' 'S'right. That's what you said I should do, wasn't it?' 'I said she would be of help to you, Tony.' 'Was I meant to do it for myself, then?' 'No, no – but it is curious, I grant you.' 'What is?' '. . . the way these things happen.' 'What about my insurance now, doctor?' 'I would advise you to apply to another company. I'll have to tell them what's happened when they write to me.' 'Why?' Dr Peckham narrowed his eyes at Tony. 'Come now, sir. You know the form. You sign a piece of paper allowing me to say things about your medical condition.' 'Yes but . . .' '. . . and I shall say them and you can have another medical.' 'Another medical?' interrupted Tony. 'Yes – no harm in that. You can never have too many medicals – and it keeps us old duffers in business, too.' 'There couldn't be some kind of error in this machine; like it leaked, or something like that, doctor?' 'Here – give me your arm. We'll check.'

Tony held out his arm. He felt the cuff going round and imagined it was his beautiful wife pumping up the cuff. Instantly, he felt relaxed and almost drowsy and the tension seemed to slip away as the cuff tightened. Then it relaxed and the throbbing began but he remained composed. Dr Peckham straightened up and ran a hand through his hair. 'Quite remarkable, Tony, I've never seen such a dramatic improvement in a man's condition in so short a time.' 'You're impressed then, doctor?' 'Impressed? I'm amazed. Well done, my boy! I don't quite know what's happened but I'm very pleased for you.' 'I think it's this little machine here. I don't know quite how it works but it's done the trick for me. I just want to tell you how grateful I am – and another thing . . .' 'Yes?' 'I think I'll forego the insurance deal for now. It seems to have been a lot of fuss over nothing. When it comes to the crunch, doctor, health comes first – eh?' Tony gave the older man an ear-to-ear grin. Then he picked up the pouch with the BP machine therein and left the room humming a tune under his breath. Dr Peckham could hear the first few bars. Mr Herbert was running through 'La Donna E Mobile'. A broad smile creased his face for just a moment; then he sat down and pressed his intercom button.

JAMES HENRY PITT-PAYNE

Beckenham

Hearts

Mrs Jones has a funny heart; she knows because the doctor says that is what is causing her blood pressure. Most funny hearts in the UK are caused by blood pressure; Mr Jones has not got blood pressure and is subsequently healthy. Mr Jones's father has not got blood pressure either, which is interesting because he is dead.

Mrs Jones has many neighbours with similar problems, and they still eat fish and chips every Friday. Some even have salt on their boiled eggs. The whole situation is in fact so serious and widespread that the Minister for Health himself has said so. In the surgery all these people (except of course the Health Minister) meet. They meet regularly, in order to discuss the merits of the world nowadays, and sometimes also to read the Spring 1981 edition of *Country Life*. Such reading matter comes generously from the doctors themselves each Spring – for authentic atmosphere.

This meeting-place has another important function for Mrs 0636 (this is of course not a standard dialling code for Ipswich but in fact a clever pseudonym for a particular person found wherever there are consulting rooms). She has an appointment for her angina. A little while ago she had late onset bronchial asthma – examination showed severe breath sounds emanating from the larynx and she has been successfully treated since on Placebo 100 mg bd. The waiting room is good for her because she still is not sure of her symptoms: easily rectified by a few concerned questions directed towards Mrs Jones (who really does have a funny heart). The new young trainee, having just finished his morning rounds after an exciting night on call, starts surgery. He is exhausted.

First on the list for morning surgery is Mrs 0636: she books early, often before she has decided why. One consequence of this is that the local family with suspected bubonic plague have been deferred from having an appointment. The consultation is as usual quick off the mark – the diagnosis made on first sight: significant cardiac disease with a non-pathological basis. The new young doctor tries red tablets 200 mg td (doubling the usual dose), but she has had these before for lumbago. 'Ah –' the doctor is stumped; she is not. Her husband is on grey tablets – she has tried them and they work much better than this rubbish. 'But . . . ' She thinks everything is all too much and the doctor agrees vehemently with that one. He finally cracks – and capitulates. Mrs 0636 marches out triumphantly. Legitimacy: an out-patient's appointment.

SAUL MILLER

Cardiff

The Private Clinic

Cyanosed blue, dilly dilly?
Bilious green?
Whate'er you hue, dilly dilly
You shall be seen

Roll up your sleeve, dilly dilly
Have a blood test,
Check your BP dilly dilly
And sound your chest

We'll put you right, dilly dilly,
Give you some pills,
Then let your firm, dilly dilly
Settle our bills

Curly Locks

Curly Locks, Curly Locks, wilt thou be mine?
Thou shalt not eat junk food, nor drink beer nor wine,
But do thine aerobics in catsuit of silk,
And dine upon muesli, stewed prunes and skimmed milk

Little Boy Blue

Little Boy Blue, put down that cream horn –
You've been overweight since the day you were born
Where is the boy who became such a creep?
He's under the daisies, six feet deep

Georgy Porgy

Georgy Porgy, salad and peas,
Gave up pie and ceased to tease
Now he's looking fit and slim
All the girls keep kissing him

(Alternative version for the London Borough of Camden)

Georgy Porgy stopped eating pie,
Got fed up with girls who cry,
Now he's handsome, slim and gay,
All the boys come out to play

MARIE CAMPKIN
London

Index

A-type personality 5
abbreviations, incomprehensibility
   of 27–8
'AC' problem 30
angina 5
angiograms 23
anticoagulants 6
arrhythmia 6
arteries 6
atheroma 6
atrium 7

B-type personality 7
beta-blockers 12
British Fat Slob 2–3
Brock, Lord 68–9

calcium blockers 12
cardiac arrest 7–8, 36–43, 47–51
   response to 55–6
cardiac neurosis 8
cardiac sphincter 8
cardiologists 8–9
cardio-thoracic surgeons 9, 59–60
cardiovascular examination made
   easy 25–6
cholesterol, serum 52
circulation 9
claudication 9
'collapse' 54
coronary arteries 10
coronary by-pass graft 10
coronary care units 10–11
coronary thrombosis 11
CVAs 17

dextrocardia 11
diet and heart disease 11–12
diuretics 12–13
drugs and the heart 12–13

electric blankets, hazards of 31
electrocardiography 13, 22–3, 28–35
examination gowns, problems
   associated 76–7

ghost in the machine 88–98
glossary 5–18

haemorrhage, reaction to 54–5
heart 13
   imagery associated 1–2
   transplants and the quality of life
   73–6
heart failure 14
heart valves 14
heartburn 13
housemen, cardiac recollections
   66–72
hypertension 14, 111–17
hypotension 14–15

Mahler, Gustav, medical history
   79–87
malt whisky and the quality of life 75
Muffage, Little Miss, and dietary
   fibre 4
murmurs 14, 15, 24–5, 58
myocardial infarction 15–16

nail varnish and anaesthesia 60
nighties, nylon, hazards of 31–2
nitrates 12

obesity 119

pacemakers 16
palpitations 16
private clinics 119
pulse, taking of 6

quality of life profile 72–6

sleep problems after heart
   transplants 74–5
smoking, dangers of 52
sphygmomanometer 16
Sprat, Jack, longevity 3
stethoscope 17, 18–22, 22–3, 57–8,
   61–2
stroke 17
syncope 17–18

terminology 5–17
treadmill tests 23

varicose veins 18
veins 18
ventricles 18